10/09 FAR

SOUND SLEEP, SOUND MIND

7 KEYS TO SLEEPING THROUGH THE NIGHT

Barry Krakow, M.D.

John Wiley & Sons, Inc.

Published by John Wiley & Sons, Inc., Hoboken, New Jersey
Published simultaneously in Canada

Charts on pages 18, 21, 25, 227, 240, 262, 271 by Maimonides Sleep Arts & Sciences, Ltd;
chart on pages 220–221 by A.D.A.M.

Wiley Bicentennial Logo: Richard J. Pacifico

Design and composition by Navta Associates, Inc.

The information contained in this book is not intended to serve as a replacement for professional medical advice. Any use of the information in this book is at the reader's discretion.
The author and the publisher specifically disclaim any and all liability arising directly or indirectly from the use or application of any information contained in this book. A health care
professional should be consulted regarding your specific situation.

For general information about our other products and services, please contact our Customer
Care Department within the United States at (800) 762-2974, outside the United States at
(317) 572-3993 or fax (317) 572-4002.

Wiley also publishes its books in a variety of electronic formats. Some content that appears
in print may not be available in electronic books. For more information about Wiley products, visit our web site at www.wiley.com.

Library of Congress Cataloging-in-Publication Data:

Krakow, Barry.
  Sound sleep, sound mind : 7 keys to sleeping through the night / Barry Krakow.
    p. cm.
  Includes index.
  ISBN 978-0-471-65064-5 (cloth)
 1. Sleep. 2. Insomnia. I. Title.
  RA786.K73 2007
  616.8'498—dc22

                                                                2007029060

Printed in the United States of America

10 9 8 7 6 5 4 3 2 1

To Marion Frankel Krakow, my loving mother
and a Woman of Valor

and

To my sleep patients, past, present, and future

Contents

PART SEVEN
HIGH-TECH SLEEP SOLUTIONS
Custom-Tailored Sleep Treatment

Acknowledgments

How this book ends may rest in my hands, but where it began surely came from so many sources and resources it would take another book to recount the story. The greatest resources for me prior to and during the actual writing of this book have been the works of Idries Shah. Many of my stories, images, pictures, analogies, and metaphors were derived directly from Shah's works or were inspired from regularly reading his works on Sufism. In the same vein, several works by or about Milton Erickson also inspired my approach.

I am also indebted to five psychiatrists. When they finally peeled off the shrink-wrapping, they found an internist-cum-emergency medicine physician-cum-sleep specialist. Arthur Deikman taught me that the emotional side of life is more about peeling an artichoke than an onion. Robert Kellner gave me a big helping hand into the research world of psychiatry. Joseph Neidhardt taught me about the richness of our dream worlds. Michael Hollifield and Roger Smith demonstrated for me time and again how psychodynamic therapy and cognitive-behavioral therapy fit together like a hand in a glove.

The number of scientists, researchers, physicians, psychologists, and other therapists to whom I am indebted for their pioneering work in the new field of sleep medicine rises into the hundreds. I want to thank Wolfgang Schmidt-Nowara, Christian Guilleminault, and Kingman Strohl for their special mentoring and support of my work.

I am also appreciative of the work of many in the field of mental health, most of whom I have not had the pleasure of meeting, but whose research greatly influenced my understanding of the connections between sleep and anxiety, depression, and posttraumatic stress.

I am also deeply indebted to many colleagues whose diligent work in and support of our clinical and research programs at the University of New Mexico School of Medicine and now at the Sleep & Human Health Institute enabled me to enhance my skills as a sleep medicine physician and researcher. Special thanks to Sharon and Teddy D. Warner, and to Dominic Melendrez, the former associate clinical and research director of our sleep programs. Much of the material in this book, including many of the questionnaires, are a direct outgrowth of my discussions about and my work in sleep medicine with Dominic, who now is advancing our field through his own company, Quality Sleep Solutions, Inc.

I also wish to thank many individuals who read various parts of the manuscript, with special gratitude to Fritz Eberle, Bruce Mann, and Chuck Paine.

I am grateful for the enduring support I received from my agents Kim Witherspoon and Alexis Hurley at InkWell Management and appreciate the patience of John Wiley & Sons. Special thanks go to my editor, Christel Winkler.

I am beholden to the CEO of our new sleep center, Maimonides Sleep Arts & Sciences, for her efforts and dedication. Although it turned into a forty-five-year global search to find and propose the job to her, the inspiration, sacrifices, and commitment provided to me by my wife, Jessica Kohr Krakow, have made all things possible.

And for Jacoby and Sable, thanks for engaging in and putting up with Daddy's incessant questions and discussions on sleep and dreams. Your input has been invaluable, and your insights will help many people sleep the good sleep.

Keys to Assessment and Monitoring Tools

Four tools help you to evaluate your sleep difficulties or monitor your treatment progress.

Sleep Misery Index, page 25
Use the index to start measuring sleep quality. Learn to link the harmful impact of insomnia and sleep quality problems on your memory and concentration, mood and emotions, energy level and day-to-day functioning.

Human Emotion Quiz, page 145
Use the quiz to learn common misconceptions and myths about feelings and emotions that plague insomniacs and other troubled sleepers. The twenty-one questions prepare you for healthier ways to work through emotions that disrupt your sleep.

Sleep-Disordered Breathing Scale, page 227
Use the scale to discover whether you suffer from a sleep breathing problem, a condition remarkably common in insomniacs and mental health patients as well as in other sleep patients. The scale also helps track improvement as treatment progresses.

PAP Therapy Follow-up Form, page 271
Use this form to monitor your response to Positive Airway Pressure (PAP) therapy, the gold standard treatment for sleep breathing problems. This treatment, also known as CPAP ("C" for Continuous), may cure your insomnia and produce the quality of sleep you might never have dreamed possible.

Introduction

The Problem: Sleeping with a Monster

What you must know right now and what you must not forget is something you may have never been told before: bad and broken sleep is never harmless!

Broken sleep must not be confused with the problem of too little sleep, popularized by an ill-informed media and misunderstood by an inattentive medical profession. The "not enough sleep" chant is all too often a cover, behind which hides a devious monster that eats away at your sleep all night long. Every night the monster attacks, some nights worse than others but always relentlessly, breaking up your sleep into little pieces. The attack fractures your sleep and destroys your ability to gain the restorative slumber you need to preserve your mental and physical health. Yet, this bad and broken sleep is nearly undetectable to every sense you possess.

Many knowledgeable people who might help you spot the monster fall for its deception, which tricks them and persuades you to think the biggest sleep problem is lack of sleep.

You must know the monster to slay it, which means recognizing that lack of sleep is only the surface of the problem.

This monster strikes deeper; it strikes at the core of your being to wound your mind, cripple your heart, and steal your breath away while robbing you of the essence of your sleep and your energy along with it. With great cunning, its all-out attack on your mind destroys your mental and emotional capacity to see this onslaught. Eventually the stealth attack on your senses from this nearly invisible sleep monster infects your life with a festering pessimism that thwarts all efforts at recovery.

Bad and broken sleep is never harmless!

The Solution: Sleep Dynamic Therapy

Sleep Dynamic Therapy (SDT) transforms this pessimism into a vigorous optimism, showing you how to sleep soundly all through the night, night after night to get the sleep you really need. From the stronger mental and physical health that follows, you reap untold rewards that can change your life.

SDT, offered in seven parts, comprises seven key principles:

1. Sleep problems are almost always sleep quality problems.
2. Changing your thoughts about sleep changes your sleep.
3. Imagery in your mind's eye is the most powerful tool you possess to put you to sleep when you want to sleep.
4. Learning to identify and cope with your feelings and emotions is the best long-term remedy for insomnia.
5. New ways to work with thoughts, feelings, and images are so powerful, you can often eliminate sleeping pills, even if currently dependent on them.
6. Unexpected physical sleep disorders, particularly those caused by problematic breathing or leg movements, affect the vast majority of troubled sleepers, especially those who insist that mental or psychological factors are the only causes.
7. Using advanced, high-tech, scientific tools and treatments, you can achieve a state of sleep the likes of which you might never have dreamed possible.

Sleep issues are almost always a matter of mind and body for both adults and children. By treating the mind and body, you will experience *Sound Sleep* and the *Sound Mind* that follows.

Throughout the book, you can use various questionnaires to measure your sleep problems and help monitor your progress. After each chapter, Sleep on It sections offer additional self-assessment tools, skills training, and pearls. Some chapters include Snooze Flashes delivering hot-off-the-press information about mental and physical aspects of sleep problems; and you'll find more news you can use on our blog at www.sleepdynamictherapy.com.

Welcome to the Sleep Dynamic Therapy program.

As you will learn, we don't take sleep problems lying down.

ALL SLEEP IS NOT THE SAME

The Sleep Quality Cure

Sleeping Happily Ever After

If a magic sleep wand were waved over your head, and you experienced *Sound Sleep* tonight, you would not need to read part one. Just one night of healthy slumber would be so enlightening, you would put every bit of energy into the quest for sound sleep. Nothing would stand in your way, because it feels so good to get the sleep you really need.

Sorry to say, all the magic wands are on back order; but don't despair, part one teaches you the arts and the sciences to change the way you see your sleep problems and to jump-start your treatment. Before you taste an orange, you must peel it. Part one peels away the tough skin of outdated and useless ideas about sleep that prevent you from relishing the fruits of sound sleep. This knowledge proves especially satisfying for those hungry to sleep without medications.

Skipping through this section undermines your chances of solving your sleep problems because you must first learn a "new language" to finally understand why you are not sleeping well or through the night. Learning this new language makes clear that a cure is truly possible.

This new language is Sleep Dynamic Therapy. Learning a language takes time, interest, and an open mind. Do you have time to learn to lay your sleep problems to rest?

It will take far less time than all the hours of lost sleep from the past year.

1

Discovering the New Sleep Medicine

Sleep Nots

All sleep is *not the same*.

There is *Sound Sleep*, in which you sleep well and through the night, night after night, and feel great every morning with energy to spare the remainder of the day . . . and there is everything else.

Sound sleep is a blessing that enriches your health and humanity. Surprisingly few people experience sound sleep; fewer genuinely appreciate the good fortune with which they are blessed; and fewer still truly understand the meaning and experience of sound sleep.

Most problematic sleepers do not realize sound sleep is their ultimate goal. How could they, since most troubled sleepers are not sure what to call their sleep problems? Many acknowledge sleep concerns, complaints, issues, difficulties, problems, disturbances, or disorders. Yet for some poor souls, sleep is so broken, it destroys their capacity to see that it's broken. Regardless of the way the problem is pictured, few grasp the true nature of sound sleep and the need to strive for it.

Most gauge sleep by hours slept, because they measure sleep in the dimension of time. If your goal is sound sleep, you must learn to measure sleep in broader and deeper dimensions, because one hour of bad or broken sleep does not equal one hour of good sleep. In fact, one hour of bad sleep barely equals thirty minutes of good sleep.

Sleep Dynamic Therapy (SDT) preaches that "all sleep is *not* the same," because this truth sets you on a path to focus on the most important question you must answer to gain sound sleep every night:

What causes your sleep difficulties?

Don't waste your efforts describing your sleep problems. Whatever your sleep concerns or complaints might be, these details can wait. To the best of your knowledge:

What are the reasons you are not getting the sound sleep you really need?

What causes you to not sleep well or all through the night, night after night, and feel great every morning, with energy to spare the remainder of the day? While many ideas come to mind, most individuals struggle with the question, and their uncertainty leads them to declare, "Hey, you're the sleep doc, you tell me!"

Minding the Body

Let's narrow the question to something about insomnia, a word meaning you have poor sleep or you are not sleeping when you want to sleep (unwanted sleeplessness). Insomnia often includes both poor sleep and not sleeping when you want to. Throughout this book, the terms "insomnia," "poor sleep," "unwanted sleeplessness," "troubled sleeper," or "problematic sleeper" are used interchangeably, because individuals with sleep problems relate to one if not all of them.

Here is a more precise "cause" question: Is your poor sleep caused by something mental (in the mind) or physical (in the body)?

Most with sleep issues select one or the other element (mental or physical) as the bigger factor. However, when sleep patients ask me, "Do you think my sleep problems are mental or physical?" my candid reply is, "Yes."

Both mind and body cause your sleep problems. Yet most with sleep difficulties dwell on something only in the mind or only in the body. This either-or perspective reflects a half-truth. Critical to your efforts is the need to move beyond this "mind or body" myth—a myth so misleading that when a person believes sleep problems could be caused by only one or the other factor (mental or physical), she will struggle in vain to solve her sleep problems and rarely achieve sound sleep.

Please take another moment—a sincere, reflective one—to reconsider your viewpoint: what do you emphasize when you think about your sleep problems? The psychological or mental factors, or the physiological or physical ones?

The best solutions treat mind and body. SDT asks you to absorb this key principle as rapidly as possible.

Quality, Not Quantity

When you apply mind-body principles of SDT, you realize that concerns about number of hours slept pale in comparison to *the real monster— Poor Sleep Quality.*

Poor sleep quality occurs almost invisibly night after night, year after year, so you cannot easily detect its impact on your sleep or your mental and physical health. Poor sleep quality is the opposite of sound sleep. When you suffer from poor sleep quality:

- You do not sleep well or all through the night, night after night.
- You do not feel great when you awaken in the morning.
- You do not have energy to spare the remainder of the day.
- You are not getting the sleep you need.

Poor sleep quality is the major cause of your sleep problems, and it determines the number of hours you sleep each and every night, whether you sleep too much or too little. Fix your sleep quality problems, and you'll almost always receive the right number of hours of sleep. In contrast, a sleep quantity yardstick does not measure sleep quality, just as a thermometer cannot measure air quality.

Some night you might sleep eight hours, but if your sleep quality were disrupted throughout the night (without your knowing it), these eight hours amount to only four, five, or six hours of sleep—very different than the eight you imagined receiving.

If you realized you slept only four hours, how would you feel the next day? Quite different than how you would feel after sleeping eight solid hours without disruption.

Poor sleep quality causes a major discrepancy between the number of hours you think you receive (clock hours) and the number of hours of good quality sleep you really obtain (solid hours). Some sleeping pills only deliver more clock hours without adding much in solid hours of sleep.

Solid Hours of Sleep is another term for *Sound Sleep.*

Once sleep quality is repaired, regardless of whether you currently sleep too little or too much, the actual number of hours you count by the clock may increase or decrease or remain unchanged in comparison to your old way of sleeping. Eventually, *clock* hours should equal *solid* hours of sleep.

SDT appreciates most troubled sleepers' keen interests in sleeping more hours. This program gently moves you toward a new perspective to gain more solid hours of sleep.

Closing In on Sleep

The monster of poor sleep quality has a treacherous daytime ally, closure problems: the inability to turn your motor to a low and smooth idle as you try to fall or stay asleep. Closure usually occurs after a reasonably satisfying waking period prior to sleep. The mind and body engage in sufficient mental, emotional, physical, and spiritual activities while awake to produce enough satisfaction to close out the day. Yet many troubled sleepers suffer difficulties in at least one of these realms.

For mental factors, best examples are unwanted thinking, such as racing thoughts or ruminations at bedtime or during the night if awakened. This inability to turn the mind from an active to a receptive mode is the single most commonly reported cause of insomnia. Instead of gradually decreasing the silent verbalizing of thoughts, self-talk, or mindless chatter, poor sleepers fret, worry, plan, or relive their dissatisfying day. This chatter is often chaotic but is sometimes fueled by exciting, upcoming events.

For emotional factors, best examples are unpleasant feelings such as anxiety or fear at bedtime or during the night if awakened. A lack of emotional closure is often the single greatest barrier to sleep, because many troubled sleepers do not know how to recognize and manage their emotions during the daytime. Anxiety is the most common emotion troubled sleepers wrestle with near bedtime, but they may not realize its presence or even call it anxiety. Restless, antsy, tense, or unsettled feelings also frequently prevent sleep.

For physical factors, best examples are physical discomfort or problematic breathing at bedtime or during the night. This lack of closure is the most deceptive, because so few troubled sleepers emphasize the physical side of their sleep complaints unless they are in pain. Yet several diagnosable, physical sleep disorders related to sleep breathing or sleep movements are common in troubled sleepers, including mental health patients.

For spiritual factors, best examples are the absence of faith, hope, or some assurance in the meaning of life. At bedtime or in the middle of the night, you feel lonely or isolated, which prevents sleep. This lack of closure may require years to understand and treat. Trauma survivors who suffer horrific events report that the meaning of life has been ripped out of their souls. In the vacuum, hopelessness, isolation, and alienation rush in. While these feelings could all be due to a mental health process, such as depression or posttraumatic stress disorder, these traumatizing events cause one to rethink one's life, irrespective of mental health problems. Sometimes the shock proves useful because it redirects one's life in new and more meaningful ways, but for many troubled sleepers the shock leaves them feeling empty and stuck. At bedtime these feelings cause enough pain to drive some survivors to suicidal thinking, a dire state magnified by poor sleep quality.

Close Calls

Closure troubles show up most glaringly as difficulty falling asleep or difficulty staying asleep and more subtly as difficulty obtaining restful sleep. Poor sleep quality further erodes the capacity of your mind and body to switch from the "active" to the "idling" position—the process of closure. Once closure problems become entrenched in your daily or nightly routines, they aggravate sleep quality problems, which then worsen closure problems, and so on in a vicious cycle.

Most problematic sleepers can spot areas of closure affecting their sleep, but few understand:

- how these factors cause sleep disturbances;
- why these factors develop;
- what is needed to gain closure.

Your relationship to time represents the best example of closure problems. Problematic sleepers routinely damage sleep through time-monitoring behaviors:

- checking the time when going to sleep;
- checking the time in the middle of the night;
- counting up hours slept if awakened at night;
- worrying about how much sleep time is left if awakened at night;
- worrying about total hours slept;
- feeling frustrated, angry, or afraid about time not slept;
- checking the clock frequently during the day;
- frequent feelings that the "clock is ticking";
- wondering how much time is left on the Big Clock.

If you had a nickel for every time . . .

Time is inextricably linked to poor sleep and to the use of sleeping pills; therefore SDT attempts to break the time barrier as the first therapeutic step to help problematic sleepers regain control over closure problems. Nearly all chronic insomnia patients and most poor sleepers enhance their slumber by breaking the lock time holds over their sleep. Indeed, as the only exception to the original advice, if you are in desperate need to improve your insomnia and you are a clock watcher, you may benefit right now by reading chapters 7 through 10 after you complete this first chapter.

Learning to Sleep Poorly

Most troubled sleepers struggle to break the time barrier not only because it is a complex closure issue, but also because time monitoring takes on a life of its own and becomes a self-defeating learned behavior that promotes poor sleep habits. The behavior develops with all the best intentions of monitoring your sleep problems, but thinking about time feeds the monster by inducing you to worry about time and sleep. Your worries worsen closure problems, because now you are thinking about lost time and lost sleep, instead of sleeping. Eventually time monitoring leads to a chronic learned behavior that breaks up your sleep quality.

Self-defeating, learned behaviors add more fuel to the cycle of sleeplessness, while sleep quality problems and closure problems conspire, through assorted mental and physical factors, to train you to be a lousy sleeper without your realizing you are learning to do so.

The surest way to solve sleep problems is to target these three critical components:

- poor sleep quality;
- closure issues;
- self-defeating, learned behaviors.

Stress and Light Sleep Myths

Tens of millions of problematic sleepers believe stress (presumably a mental thing) or being a light sleeper (presumably a physical thing) is to blame for insomnia or poor sleep. They declare, "I'm just stressed out" or "I'm a light sleeper."

While these perceptions are offered earnestly, they reflect half-truths because stress and light sleep rarely if ever turn out to be the whole explanation for anyone's sleep problems.

Show me an individual with insomnia who claims her problem is stress, and SDT uncovers at least five more important mental and physical factors underlying her unwanted sleeplessness. Show me a poor sleeper who claims his problem is light sleep, and SDT uncovers five more important mental and physical factors underlying his light slumber.

Stress and light sleep are worth investigating, but these terms function as buzz words that distract you from the mind-body approach required to solve 95 percent of sleep disturbances. Some troubled sleepers use these expressions to avoid discussing sleep problems altogether. SDT shows how stress and light sleep fit into a broader framework that will more clearly explain your sleep problems.

Starting Fresh

Despite overwhelming scientific evidence that sleep is one of the most critical human health functions in which we must engage, and that poor sleep damages and prematurely ages our minds, bodies, and ultimately our spirits, physicians and therapists remain largely unaware of how sound sleep improves mental and physical health. Worse, many health-care professionals, working with the best intentions, do not recognize the vicious cycle triggered by poor sleep quality, closure problems, and learned poor sleep habits. Many discount or minimize patients' sleep problems. A large percentage of health-care providers assume sleep problems concern number of hours slept, which explains their reliance on incomplete therapies such as prescription or nonprescription medications and simplistic sleep tips. As most health-care practitioners have no formal background, training, or experience in the burgeoning field of sleep disorders medicine, their treatments may yield weak, inconsistent, and sometimes dangerous results.

I do not seek to demean the character or intent of health-care professionals, most of whom are hardworking and dedicated to their patients. And I apologize to any practitioner who might misinterpret my views. Sleep medicine is a new field for most health-care workers, so sleep complaints routinely fall below the radar, which leads to incomplete evaluation and treatment.

The objective is to warn you about the influence of your past treatment experiences, which might interfere with learning about mind-body sleep medicine perspectives. What if you previously sought help from a doctor who did not take your sleep complaints seriously? What if you asked for assistance from a mental health professional who believed the only way to fix your sleep problem was to first fix your psychiatric problem? What if you received imprecise advice from a doctor or a therapist and found it relatively useless or ineffective?

Such experiences are common. Beyond demonstrating little respect for sleep problems, these encounters provoke annoyance, frustration, or possibly anger, embarrassment, or shame among those seeking answers to real health problems. Predictably, many troubled sleepers wind up reading superficial suggestions from newspaper or magazine articles that rarely solve anyone's sleep problems, while some individuals never seek assistance, because they imagine nothing could possibly help. Some depend on sleeping pills or other substances, which often feel about as satisfying as showering with your clothes on.

Whatever the nature of these prior experiences, you must determine whether they foster confusion or skepticism about treating sleep problems, and whether they bias you against mind-body perspectives. Now is the time to start with a fresh perspective.

The Great Divide

How does a mind-body connection strike you?

Our society's current medical emphasis on separating mental and physical factors instead of combining them (mind-body medicine) is deeply ingrained in our history; our culture; and, unfortunately, our sciences. This tendency springs from a curious belief that the mind and the body are distinct things, operating in unrelated ways, as if the words to a song and its melody were unconnected. Despite the near universal preference to think about one's health with an "either-or" (mental or physical) attitude, the mind and the body are inseparable and always act in concert. Although it takes time to appreciate this health perspective, it can never be overemphasized.

You may believe that stress or mental health concerns are the only explanations for your troubled sleep. Among the several thousand such problematic sleepers seeking treatment at our centers, most had attempted every form of stress reduction, psychotherapy, or taken every sort of sleeping pill, tranquilizer, antidepressant, or mood stabilizer, yet rarely did these therapies conquer their sleeplessness. Whereas, when we treated the physical components of their insomnia, they made dramatic improvements, and some achieved a genuine cure.

Our sleep centers also have worked with thousands of problematic sleepers convinced that light sleep and physical factors were the only causes of their troubled sleep. Most had tried every sort of physical treatment, such as breathing devices for sleep breathing problems or medications for leg movement conditions, yet they, too, did not achieve the desired results. Whereas, when we treated mental components of poor sleep, they made dramatic improvements, and some achieved a complete cure.

Divorcing mind and body rarely produces long-term health solutions; whereas, respecting the holy matrimony of mind and body guides you to dramatic improvements in sleep, if not outright cures.

Dynamic Solutions

Every night, your mind and your body need a break from the world; you deserve that break. In both small and large ways, SDT teaches you how to gain the *rest of your life*.

It should go without saying that you would visit a neurosurgeon for a brain tumor or a cardiologist for heart disease, but few of our medical and mental health colleagues send patients regularly to sleep medicine specialists. Even fewer health-care providers recognize the need to address sleep complaints with a mind-body approach.

For these reasons, you are well served now to know that SDT does not offer a bunch of tips, shortcuts, or quick fixes to solve your sleep problems; it is not a "book for dummies," because the average sleep patient has intelligence far above average. It's not a book for someone who imagines he can learn to speed-read poetry. Reading poetry, just like reading your sleep problems, takes time and requires a fresh mind-set, one in which you learn to think, to feel, and to see things in a new light. SDT shines a uniquely brighter light on your sleep problems, so that when you turn off the lights, you can sleep soundly through the night and get the sleep you really need.

In the next five chapters, you start a transforming process by learning how mind and body are wedded to each other. With this knowledge, you will work on mental causes of sleep problems, while realizing you are improving physical aspects of sleep as well. And as you work on physical causes, you improve mental aspects of sleep, too.

The Journey Begins

SDT requires an open mind and a willingness to attempt suggestions and instructions that follow. In this new sleep treatment program, rest assured you will find many solutions to your personal sleep issues.

If concerns, doubts, or motivation issues persist, consider the woman who woke up each day eager to make a delicious omelet with tasty vegetables and flavorful spices. Regrettably, when she finished her cooking, she always ended up with a bowl of glop and a lost appetite. The wrong ingredients and the wrong recipe sealed her fate, because no one ever showed her the right stuff to put in the frying pan or how to cook it.

Few health-care professionals outside the field of sleep medicine recognize the special ingredients required for healthy slumber. Fewer still know how to craft a recipe to resolve sleep disorders. To succeed, you must know the mental and physical elements (proper ingredients) that promote sound sleep. And you must adopt a comprehensive treatment strategy (best recipe) through which you can regularly obtain *Sound Sleep* and the *Sound Mind* that will awaken refreshed and ready to take on the day each and every morning.

Now you will learn how to do just that.

The Sleep on It Assessment Program

Few people receive knowledge by pouring it in as if they were an empty vessel. Most approach learning with a full tank, overflowing with ideas on the very thing they want to learn about. This analogy reflects the paradox in learning about sleep problems. Although you possess a strong desire for help, you also have opinions about your sleep problems, some of which could interfere with your ability to learn new concepts.

Pouring large volumes of information into a full tank makes a mess. A more prudent approach mixes a little of the new stuff with the old stuff. In virtually all fields of learning, the tastiest mixture is brewed by offering challenging questions in a friendly, stimulating, and curious way. This technique engages you to think and rethink things until the new information is thoroughly digested.

At the close of each chapter, questions are posed to stimulate your curiosity and spark your desire:

- to gain new insights about sleep disturbances;
- to help you develop skills to use various treatment steps;
- to use practical instructions to solve your sleep problems.

Each Question is followed by a Comment and then a Pearl.

SLEEP ON IT
The Mind-Body Connection

QUESTION: In your mind's eye, picture a pie and divide it into two portions. One portion represents the mental side of your sleep problem and the other portion represents the physical side. "To thine own self be true" makes a world of difference in solving sleep problems, so start your sleep therapy by candidly informing yourself about these portions, even though they may change. Measuring two slices by percentages (for example, 75 percent mental and 25 percent physical, 50–50, or 10–90) are ways to slice it.

Please jot down your percentages here:

Mental   = _____ %
Physical = _____ %
Total   =   100%

COMMENT: Most people with sleep problems, especially those with mental health symptoms such as anxiety, depression, or posttraumatic stress, believe that their sleep difficulties are about mental factors and often mark down 90 percent in the mental category and only 10 percent in the physical. Most people with insomnia believe that mental stress is the leading or the only cause as well. Few problematic sleepers hear much to challenge this mental perspective.

Now you will be challenged—because a predominant mental view of sleep disturbances is a great myth that we must dispel as politely but as urgently as possible—so you more naturally think in terms of a 50–50 relationship between psychological and physiological sleep factors.

Perhaps you've wondered whether physical factors were lurking behind the more obvious mental components of your sleep problems. Now would be the time to explore your theories.

――――― PEARL ―――――
Watching the Clock Is Bad Medicine

Surely, these ideas are something to sleep on, and nothing will move you in this direction faster than recognizing how your psychological attitudes about time actually help or harm the physiology of your sleep. Time may march on, but don't let it stomp all over your sleep quality. As you will learn in part two— chapters 7 through 10, the first section on treatment—when it comes to sleep, time is never of the essence!

2

Building a Sleep Quality Brain Trust

The Brain Reigns

Understanding brain activity during rest or sleep gives you the confidence to trust the 50–50, mind-body perspective on poor sleep quality.

Consider rest. You move your body into a comfortable position that requires no effort to maintain. You try to slow or stop certain activities in your mind and your body. Your limbs and torso relax so that most muscles work minimally. Your mind quiets down as you daydream or watch a relaxing program on television. At this point, you might guess you achieved a state of rest.

Guess again. Rest emerges only when your body responds with additional physiological changes. Your heart rate and breathing rate must decrease, and usually your temperature drops, too, because blood flow increases to the hands and the feet, releasing more heat through the skin. These physical changes must occur for rest to be restful. The absence of physical changes explains why some insomnia patients do not improve with relaxation techniques. Their heart rate, depth of breathing, or temperature may not change to produce a restful state; and, adding insult to injury, an insomniac lying awake in bed in the middle of the night is not only not sleeping but also not resting.

The key to rest is not just inactivity. Physiological functions of the body must respond as well, and the brain makes or prevents these changes from happening.

As in rest, similar changes occur with sleep. The brain instructs you to find a comfortable position for the body that requires minimal effort to maintain, and it limits unnecessary mental and physical activity. At times throughout sleep, the brain takes advantage of the picture show in your mind's eye—dreaming—to catch up and reassess recent waking experiences or rehearse future events, all without lifting a finger, even when you change channels. Again, the brain must conform to sleep physiology and produce changes in heart rate, breathing rate, and blood flow to achieve restorative slumber. Without these changes, sleep quality is nonrestorative.

Nowhere are these changes more evident than in the brain waves, because if they do not decrease in activity, physiological functions cannot change either.

Quality Squiggles

A wondrous thing about the mind-body is that physiological activity can be measured to determine how well one rests or sleeps. In a sleep laboratory, brain waves—known as electroencephalographic or EEG patterns—are measured by attaching electrodes to the scalp. The recorded nerve signals are converted into squiggly lines on a piece of paper or computer display. These brain waves run in a continuous sequence, like a row of up-and-down lines, as if drawn by a pen held in a shaky hand that never lifts the point off the paper—picture a doctor's scribble, slightly more legible (chart 1).

The naked eye can easily spot when brain waves speed up or slow down. As you expect, brain waves cycle faster while awake, consistent with increased activity, both mental and physical. When brain waves slow down, you could be resting, meditating, or sleeping. Within sleep, a range of brain wave activity appears, usually based on three broad types of sleep. These types correspond to five biological sleep stages:

- deeper, or delta, sleep: corresponds to nonrapid-eye-movement (NREM) stage 3 or 4 sleep;
- lighter sleep: corresponds to nonrapid-eye-movement (NREM) stage 1 or 2 sleep;
- dream awareness sleep: corresponds to rapid-eye-movement (REM) sleep.

Deep sleep generates the slowest brain wave activity: the squiggly lines on the computer screen go up and down more slowly and look less dense. You see white space between lines, because they take as much as a half to

Chart 1. Basic Sleep Stages in a Normal Sleeper

A. Awake

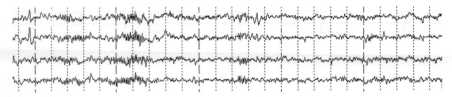

B. Stage 2 NREM

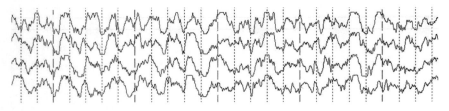

C. Delta Sleep

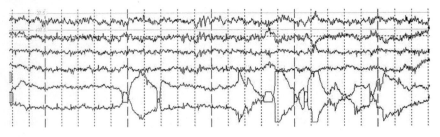

D. Rapid-Eye-Movement (REM) Sleep

Each graph spans thirty seconds, and the first four tracing lines represent brain waves (EEG) detected by sensors attached to the head. (A). Brain waves while awake are faster than sleep brain waves and therefore look denser. (B). Stage 2 NREM is the most common sleep stage, accounting for as much as 50 percent or more of sleep. While the amplitude (height) of the wave is similar to awake brain waves, notice how its slower frequency creates more white space in the picture. (C). Delta sleep is the most restorative stage of sleep, and the waves are the least dense and the slowest. Adults average about 10 to 15 percent of the night in delta. (D). REM sleep, named for the rapid movements of the eyes in various directions, is shown in the two eye channels below the brain wave channels. In some ways the brain waves look similar to both wake and stage 2 NREM. Although we dream in all stages of sleep, most people have more awareness of dreams occurring in REM.

a whole second to go up and down. These taller and wider squiggles are delta waves and correspond to your most restorative sleep.

Lighter sleep is restorative, but stage 2 NREM generates faster and therefore shorter, narrower waveforms, sometimes as fast as fifteen sets of up-and-down squiggles in a single second. This sleep looks denser, but you still rest because lighter stages produce brain wave activity slower than waking activity. Even so, there is no comparison to how a person feels when he or she receives more stage 3 or 4 NREM versus stage 2 NREM. The deeper stages are more refreshing, and virtually any sleeper detects this difference.

Pause for a moment and appreciate that we just described the brain's nervous system activity and appearance during sleep. Although squiggly lines represent the work of millions of nerve cells generating billions of impulses, an EEG draws a gross but useful picture of the sleep process, which yields a relatively consistent measure of sleep quality. In a nutshell, when the brain speeds up during sleep, quality goes down. When brain waves remain rhythmical or consolidated and keep a slower pace consistent for each sleep stage, quality goes up.

Slower EEG = good sleep quality.

Faster EEG = poor sleep quality.

To solve your sleep problems, keep these waves in mind.

The Brain in Action

While waveforms are influenced by mental factors, there can be no denying that they involve a physical component. If you find a way to slow down your brain waves, much of your human physiology slows down as well while your sleep quality goes up.

REM sleep is somewhat unusual, because the pattern combines assorted waveforms that fluctuate above or below the frequencies of lighter sleep stages. The speeds of REM brain waves alternate between faster or slower rates compared to rates in NREM light sleep. But REM sleep is still restorative when it is consolidated.

The measure of sleep consolidation in any stage means how long you remain in a particular stage of sleep with a rhythmical flow of brain waves uninterrupted by other influences. If you toss and turn a lot during sleep, each movement speeds up your brain and interrupts the rhythmical flow of waveforms. Technically you arouse or actually awaken during this movement, destroying your consolidation. Many troubled sleepers toss and turn a lot, and most assign stress, worry, or other mental factors as the cause. Some say they just can't get comfortable, which they link to a mental process such as racing thoughts.

Granted, all these points are relevant, but your body is still moving! And sleep brain waves change with every toss and turn, pushing you out of a state of sound sleep into one of poor sleep quality. Thus poor sleep quality is a decidedly physical, measurable, and fixable problem. And nowhere is poor sleep quality more evident in a sleep lab, where this problem frequently manifests as too much time spent in stage 1 NREM. Remarkably, this lightest of all sleep stages rarely consolidates your slumber; often, it functions like broken sleep as you cycle between waking and sleeping brain waves.

Broken Sleep

When we record brain signals in a sleep lab, we look closely for things that interfere with natural sleep consolidation (chart 2). Literally, we want to measure how much your sleep is broken.

This fragmenting pattern of interruptions, inconsistent with high-quality slumber, includes:

- awakenings, lasting 15 seconds or longer;
- arousals, lasting 3 to 15 seconds;
- microarousals, lasting 1.5 to 3 seconds;
- transitions between wakefulness and sleep;
- overall, too much lighter sleep, stage 1 NREM;
- short, broken-up periods of delta or REM sleep;
- excessive physical movements of various muscles (for example, in chin or legs).

Each of these patterns is too fast or too active to consolidate into deeper or higher-quality sleep. In contrast, *Sound Sleep* looks slower, quieter, and more consolidated because the fragmenting patterns described above are absent; whereas poor sleep quality looks faster, noisier, and fragmented. In sleep lab jargon, these distinctions are summarized with the two terms we've been using:

- Consolidation = a reflection of good sleep quality.
- Fragmentation = a reflection of poor sleep quality.

Even during REM sleep, wherein every sleeper's brain is more active (potentially faster brain waves), EEG is still more consolidated during

Chart 2. Sleep Fragmentation

A. Microarousal

B. Arousal

C. Awakening

D. Stage 1 NREM

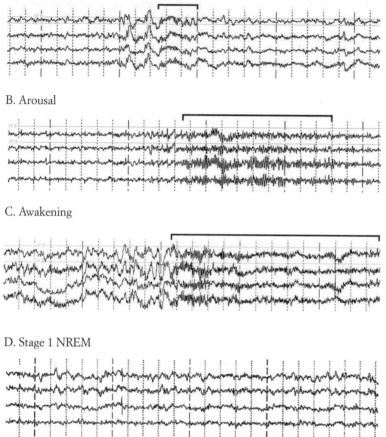

Each graph spans thirty seconds, and the four tracing lines represent brain waves (EEG) detected by sensors attached to the head. At the start of each of the first three graphs, the EEG shows sleep, then the brain waves speed up (bracketed area) and look more dense or darker. These denser brain waves reflect a state that is close to or actually awake, and this speeding up process in the middle of sleep destroys healthy sleep consolidation. The result is broken sleep, our term for physiological sleep fragmentation. (A). Microarousal. The smallest of the measurable forms of arousal; it usually lasts 1.5 to 3 seconds. (B). Arousal. These are the most common arousals seen in patients suffering from significant sleep fragmentation. They measure between 3 and 15 seconds. (C). Awakening. These patterns look like arousals, but they are longer than 15 seconds, and thus are technically deemed an awakening. The sleeper might return readily to sleep or awaken for several minutes or longer. Awakening is a misnomer, because few sleepers remember being awake unless they are awake for more than 5 minutes. (D). Stage 1 NREM sleep. As you will learn, this lightest stage of sleep is a fundamental part of sleep fragmentation. When sleep is broken, it frequently alternates between wakefulness and stage 1 sleep.

sound sleep. However, in someone with poor sleep quality, brain waves in REM sleep often exhibit the worst forms of fragmentation.

What causes all this broken sleep is a major controversy in our field of sleep medicine. Some research supports the view that chronic insomnia patients suffer lighter sleep as innate sleep fragmentation due to frequent "spontaneous arousals," when the brain waves speed up for no apparent reason. Our research team has long held that these arousals may not be spontaneous but instead could be caused by other physical factors, such as breathing or movement disorders. The one thing that all agree on is that sleep fragmentation, from whatever cause, compromises sleep quality and leads to poor health in more ways than you would imagine.

Broken Sleep Is Never Harmless

When sleep fragmentation patterns persist for years or decades, other physiological systems that should be resting also become fragmented or adversely affected. Both heart rate and blood pressure increase during or after certain types of sleep fragmentation; and it is clear that sleep fragmentation caused by sleep breathing problems is linked to cardiovascular disease, including heart attacks, strokes, heart rhythm disturbances, congestive heart failure, and cardiac chest pain. More recently, broken sleep has been shown to worsen blood sugar control.

Equally dramatic are the short-run consequences of sleep fragmentation, which also produce many different symptoms in your mental and physical health, yet you might find it impossible to believe all these connections to broken sleep. Before you confront this list of ill effects, first consider the ultimate purpose of sleep, which should make it much easier to appreciate the wallop delivered by the frazzled brain waves of sleep fragmentation.

Sleep Dividends

Investing in sound sleep is one of the safest, most durable health strategies. Nightly, high-quality deposits of slumber into your sleep bank account will not only last a lifetime, but they also have a clear potential to increase your life span. In simplest terms, the capacity of the brain to slow itself down (sleeping) serves to restore, regenerate, and revitalize your mind and body nightly; without sleep, your mind and body degenerate. And in experiments with rats, total sleep deprivation caused their death.

Sleep also aids most healing processes and prevents all sorts of ailments that afflict your mental and physical health by strengthening your immune system and effectively repairing other systems in your body. Night after night of sound sleep is saving your life over and over again; whereas night after night of broken sleep is killing you off, slowly but surely.

When your sleep is of a higher quality, you experience fewer infections and accidents, less risk for mental illness such as depression, and less risk for physical illness such as heart disease. Yet if you suffer from any of these conditions, you seem to recover from them faster, or at least achieve greater improvements, when you regularly obtain sound sleep during the healing stages.

Good-quality sleep is very good for your heart and the rest of your cardiovascular system, because sound sleep lowers your blood pressure and heart rate at night. Sleeping well also decreases your stress levels overnight and gives you more energy to cope with new stress the next day. Good sleep quality sharpens your mental functions as it enhances memory; promotes learning of new material—truly makes you smarter; and, of great interest to problematic sleepers with emotional closure issues, good sleep quality increases the capacity to work through or "process" the full range of feelings, thus enhancing mental health. In addition, sound sleep is a pleasurable human behavior, which is how those blessed with high-quality sleep describe it. Overall, sleep is something nutritious, which nourishes and repairs mind and body and satisfies you in the process.

Wholesome sleep and wholesome food share a lot in common. Without wholesome sleep, you are literally starving your mind and body of essential nutrients that enable you to think, feel, perceive, and function at your best. Worse, when you starve yourself of wholesome sleep for years or decades, your mental and physical health suffer tremendous injury and sometimes irreversible damage—damage to your heart and your brain, indisputably as bad as or worse than smoking cigarettes or drinking too much alcohol.

Sleep is a very big deal, because *Poor Sleep Quality* destroys your health, whereas *Sound Sleep* provides immeasurable health benefits to mind and body.

All sleep is not the same . . . and your brain waves provide the living proof.

At the Crossroads

Few people with sleep problems actually believe sleep has this much power over their mental and physical health. Most poor sleepers are likely to dismiss this information because it just does not register. How could sleep possibly be this important?

To which I ask, "How could sleep *not* be this important?"

We have been blessed with an incredibly complex and highly functional system, called the human mind and body. With it, we can do incredible things, such as paint, draw, sing, yodel, talk, and write. We can run, dance, skip, and jump, not to mention hop on one leg. We can engage in intensely pleasurable actions, such as making love or music, laughing, reading, and singing. We can move arms and legs to hit a golf or a tennis ball, throw a football or a baseball, kick a soccer ball, and, amazingly, we can swim across water without sinking. We can build things, invent things, create things, work on things, love things, and even procreate our species. At the end of the day, we can relive all these things through our thoughts, feelings, and images in the mind's eye.

Please tell me how something capable of this much complex action could *not* need an incredibly complex, resourceful, and efficient system to repair itself? How could we possibly be so greedy as to think the human system just gets by, that somehow our incredibly intricate operating systems just repair themselves only on the fly (which they also do all the time as well), and that no rest or restoration would ever be needed? What other organic system possesses a complexity anywhere close to humans and gets by without sleep?

There is none. And with all this complexity, we need to use only a quarter to a third of the day to maintain our systems.

You may not yet believe in sleep, but I guarantee that sleep believes in you and knows what's at stake in helping you not only to survive but also to live a balanced and prosperous life.

To repeat, sleep is a very big deal: the magnitude of sleep's impact on one's health may be as great as or greater than that of any other essential system within the human organism.

Poor Sleep Quality, therefore, is nothing short of a ticking time bomb with a long, slow fuse, whose impact directly and sometimes irreversibly harms your cardiovascular system and your nervous system as well as many other facets of your mental and physical health. Not treating your sleep problems can have serious consequences to your health, which is why SDT teaches you to take your sleep problems seriously.

To start, you must recognize that sleep quality problems in the form of fragmented brain waves drive most sleep problems. Therefore, sleep quality is the key to solving them.

. . .

This dramatic news is designed to wake you up to the realities of poor sleep. Connecting your own sleep problems to other health difficulties in your daily life is the fastest way to motivate yourself to aggressively treat your sleep complaints. There is no better way to start making these connections than to test yourself on the Sleep Misery Index.

Sleep Misery Index

	Frequency (How *often* do you have . . .)			
	Never	Sometimes	Often	Always
Cognitive/Mental Capacity				
Difficulty paying attention	☐	☐	☐	☐
Difficulty concentrating	☐	☐	☐	☐
Memory problems	☐	☐	☐	☐
Making simple mistakes	☐	☐	☐	☐
Misplacing things	☐	☐	☐	☐
Forgetting where things are	☐	☐	☐	☐
Emotional/Mood Capacity				
Anxious feelings	☐	☐	☐	☐
Irritability	☐	☐	☐	☐
Depressive feelings	☐	☐	☐	☐
Hostile or angry feelings	☐	☐	☐	☐
Easily frustrated	☐	☐	☐	☐
Decreased sexual interest or pleasure	☐	☐	☐	☐
Energy/Engagement Capacity				
Decreased activity level	☐	☐	☐	☐
Low energy	☐	☐	☐	☐
Sleepiness during the day	☐	☐	☐	☐
Chronic fatigue	☐	☐	☐	☐
Tiredness during the day	☐	☐	☐	☐
Feeling like everything's an effort	☐	☐	☐	☐
Lack of interest in things	☐	☐	☐	☐
Feeling slowed down	☐	☐	☐	☐
Feeling unproductive	☐	☐	☐	☐

SLEEP ON IT
Sleep Misery Index

QUESTION: How did you fare on the Sleep Misery Index?

COMMENT: Notice how the symptoms listed affect how you think about the world, how you feel about things in the world, how you see things in the world, and as a consequence, how you function from day to day.

The first component involves cognitive and mental impairment. Consider the problem of not remembering where you put your keys. You must pay attention or concentrate when you put your keys down. Then you have to store this experience in memory to retrieve it. Last, you must recall this information when you need your keys again. How often do you misplace your keys?

You might be stunned to realize how a simple behavior or misbehavior of this sort is directly tied to a sleep quality problem. When your brain waves are frazzled, preventing you from restoring cognitive abilities, you are bound to suffer impaired attention, concentration, or memory. As a result, you forget things and make simple mistakes in your daily life.

The second component involves the way you manage your emotions and your mood. All emotions tie into mental health concerns or outright disorders and are extremely important to evaluate when considering the strength and stability of your mind. Many emotions are adversely influenced when excessive brain wave activity at night leaves you sleepy, tired, or fatigued the next day.

When you find yourself in situations in which you are easily frustrated or angered, how often do you consider whether you are also sleepy, tired, or fatigued? Most people do not put these puzzle pieces together. They have forgotten or never learned that a tired and weary mind yields hasty and useless solutions. It is far too easy to imagine the problem as anger or perhaps too much tension from a state of perpetual frustration. While these analyses might prove valid, how often does anyone ask whether you might suffer from a short fuse due to exhaustion caused by poor sleep quality?

The third area deals with the way you manage your energy and your activity level. It includes the classic triad of sleepiness, tiredness, and fatigue as well as many elements about the way you function from day to day. When your interest wanes and everything seems like an effort, you feel slowed down and unproductive. Nowadays, depression is the first picture that might pop into your or your doctor's mind. Or you might mistake the problem for boredom.

Most troubled sleepers make no immediate connection between these symptom clusters and poor sleep quality. Many troubled sleepers sleepwalk through life, suffering dampened, pessimistic outlooks in which the potential for change rarely appears on the horizon. Most believe these symptoms are normal or normal aging, whereas some seek medication, such as antidepressants. It may look, smell, sound, feel, or even taste like depression, but sleep disorders mimic the entire experience of depression with nearly identical symptoms and intensity.

———— P E A R L ————
Rating Sleep Quality Is the Fast Track to Success

If you could link these symptoms directly to a sleep problem, you would become highly motivated to treat the problem. So how easy is it to make this link? It may seem unbelievable at this point, but the value of the Sleep Misery Index is that the symptoms are an indirect but accurate way to estimate sleep quality. Even if you are not convinced of these connections just yet, you can at least start monitoring these symptoms to see whether you can link them to the way you sleep.

More than 90 percent of readers may not yet be ready to accurately rate their own sleep quality, although I hope your desire to rate your sleep quality is mounting fast.

3

The Anti-Sandman

Removing Sleep Blinders

If you are ready to rate the quality of your sleep, move to chapter 5. However, most poor sleepers are challenged by several common barriers that distort or impair their ability to assess sleep quality. These barriers prevent you from linking broken sleep to various health consequences; and without these links, your progress is slowed. Even if you cannot overcome these barriers immediately, just spotting them keeps you headed in the right direction.

This section is tough. You will be looking into a very clear mirror, but when you finish this self-analysis, you will possess a much greater ability to rate the quality of your sleep, the most critical step to success.

Barrier 1: Out of Sight, Out of Mind

Barrier 1 requires immediate recognition and acceptance of these facts:

- You are not "present" when you sleep.
- You are not watching yourself sleep.
- You are not monitoring or measuring anything while you sleep.
- You are not listening to yourself sleep.
- Most importantly, you cannot go back and remember what happens with your actual sleep—as opposed to time awake during the night—because you were asleep at the time and have little memory of the experience, except for dreams.

Because you suffer from "amnesia" for what happens during sleep, you could be the last person in the world to depend on to reliably describe your sleep quality.

How could you possibly examine all the physical and mental components of your sleep quality when you are not there to observe anything while you sleep? How could you possibly know why you wake up in the middle of the night? You were asleep before you woke, so how could you know what awakened you?

You cannot know, so please stop trying to know until you gain sufficient information and clues to pinpoint the nature of these problems.

This barrier is only problematic if you insist on believing that you can analyze your own sleep quality directly. Once you realize there are many indirect ways during the day to assess sleep quality, you quickly ease any pressure to guess what's happening at night.

Broken Sleep Revisited

If you continue to speculate about your sleep without proper tools, chances are high you will never accept that your sleep might be broken. While rare patients show minimal signs of broken sleep, you are better off assuming that you suffer some sleep fragmentation—your sleep is breaking up into pieces, big or small, during the night. Just accepting the possibility of broken sleep frees your resources in three ways:

1. You no longer feel pressure to search for quick fixes that do not resolve sleep problems, because you accept that shortcuts do not repair broken sleep.
2. You no longer feel as much anxiety about number of hours slept, because you realize that broken sleep is the real problem causing short sleep.
3. You no longer are confused about the nature of sleep problems, because you can focus on your broken sleep and repair it.

Honestly admitting that your sleep is broken is a potent step that opens your mind to more effective treatment options and helps you overcome the out-of-sight, out-of-mind barrier.

Barrier 2: What's Really Normal?

Awareness of sleep disorders in our society has not reached the tipping point, wherein the masses fully accept sleep problems as something common and in need of treatment. In the United States, our culture belittles or ignores sleep issues, which means that whenever the topic of sleep arises—and people do talk about needing more sleep or feeling tired or sleepy during the day—the discussion serves not to educate but to normalize the experience.

It's considered okay to:

- drink four to six caffeinated beverages per day;
- be drowsy while you drive;
- struggle to get out of bed in the morning;
- get too little sleep;
- feel exhausted at various points in the day;
- feel behind schedule in your daily activities.

Why are these considered okay? Because when two thirds of Americans report problems with their sleep—which they do, but which they avoid linking to fatigue and sleepiness behaviors described above—then they think that the least threatening way to deal with this information is to assume everything's normal.

A lot of people suffer from sleep problems, but that does not make these problems normal!

Can you imagine anyone in the medical profession declaring that two thirds of all adults suffer from heart disease, hypertension, or diabetes, so we can safely assume that these conditions are normal phases of aging that don't require treatment?

Selection of these three ailments is not coincidental. As stated previously, clear evidence shows important relationships between these three deadly diseases and broken sleep due to various sleep disorders. But when was the last time your primary-care physician or therapist declared it was time for your annual sleep checkup?

Human Energy Generator

Too much talk about feeling tired or sleepy is not viewed favorably in our society. Such individuals do not appear productive, and they would not receive a reward and probably not receive sympathy for complaints of low energy due to fatigue or sleepiness. Rather, they might be ridiculed, embarrassed, or shamed. Such experiences drive many troubled sleepers, both adults and adolescents, to disregard fatigue and sleepiness or find expedient ways to make them "disappear."

A dangerous example of this "disappearing act" occurs among those who become hooked on caffeinated coffee, tea, or soda. Once an individual regularly minimizes or eliminates low energy by self-medicating with these drinks, there is virtually no chance of stopping this behavior to examine actual causes. Instead, sleepiness and fatigue "magically" disappear, while chronic sleep fragmentation persists. The danger arises because sleep disorders and their serious symptoms of fatigue and sleepiness lie in the shadows, yet still put you at risk for an array of problems, including drug use and abuse, alcoholism, car accidents, depression, suicide, and a host of medical conditions.

Few people with sleep problems link chronic caffeine use to a desire to boost energy. Few recognize anything abnormal in their excessive use of caffeine. Truly, there is a plague of fatigue and sleepiness in our land, which arguably explains the explosive growth of coffee shops in the past decade.

Ultimately, questions must be asked: Why is it so difficult to put together these puzzle pieces? Why is it so difficult to spot a malfunction in your human energy generator—the natural, physiological, human capacity to generate energy otherwise known as sleeping?

You must stop normalizing these symptoms to accurately assess your sleep quality.

Barrier 3: Sleeping Is Believing

If you have never experienced *Sound Sleep*, you don't know what you're missing, and you may be incapable of imagining a life without daytime fatigue and sleepiness. It might be too difficult to spot the connection between symptoms and sleep quality until you first resolve the problem and observe the changes. When sleep quality improves, and fatigue and sleepiness decrease or disappear, it is easier to fathom the full impact the problem had on your life and lifestyle. This "sleeping is believing" approach affects nearly everyone with sleep disorders, because it is impossible to test the waters otherwise.

Poor sleep quality is not an illness that erupts overnight; it is a chronic condition that happens every night. It gradually forms a veil over your senses, unwittingly leading you to normalize sleepiness and fatigue. The most accurate and reliable way to prove to yourself that sleep quality has moved from bad to good is to experience firsthand the feelings of not being tired, fatigued, or sleepy during the day, which is something you can grasp while awake.

Striking examples of these changes are witnessed by savvy health-care professionals who refer patients to sleep centers. Friends and family members are delighted by the dramatic changes in loved ones. These sleep patients are newly revitalized individuals who look healthier and younger, function more effectively, and communicate more clearly because they conquered their sleep quality woes and dramatically decreased their fatigue and sleepiness. Although such resoundingly positive changes are commonplace at sleep medical centers, the vast majority of problematic sleepers go to "sleep centers" to shop for mattresses.

Barrier 4: The Ultimate Mind Game

The *Sound Sleep, Sound Mind* perspective is not held by most health-care professionals despite growing evidence to support this knowledge. The twenty-first century may be out of diapers, past the toddler stage, and approaching kindergarten, but it has yet to develop a mature, intelligent perspective on the critical interrelationships between sleep and mental health. Perspectives on sleep and stress are clearer but remain flawed. These flaws, which overemphasize the importance of mental health or stress on sleep while discounting the impact of sleep on stress and mental health, serve as the most complex barriers preventing sleep patients from seeking and receiving proper sleep medical care.

Many people with sleep and mental health concerns hear or take up the chant "Take care of your mental health, and sleep will take care of itself."

This mental health slant on sleep disorders is an outdated, overly simplistic psychiatric or psychological approach that results in inadequate or incomplete care of sleep disturbances. Regrettably, the stage is set for malpractice issues to become a growing influence on the way sleep medicine is integrated into our health-care systems. Sleep specialists treat a fair number of patients who have been improperly diagnosed with mental health problems (most commonly depression) that were actually sleep disorders, or the sleep disorder was missed as it coincided with the mental disorder. Sleep specialists often hear discouraging accounts from patients who were prevented for years or decades from receiving standard sleep medicine therapies at sleep centers because their doctors or therapists declared their sleep problems mere symptoms of a mental disorder.

Sleep and mental health problems frequently reside on opposite sides of the same coin. Unfortunately, each of your physicians or therapists may see only one side. In ideal circumstances, sleep specialists and mental health professionals would build bridges toward the other's respective field, making it easier for patients to cross over into either specialty to receive the maximum therapeutic response from both sleep and mental health treatments.

This bridge will not be built overnight. Problematic sleepers must contend with the fact that sleep specialists and mental health professionals don't work together enough of the time to spawn new views about sleep problems in mental health patients, which exacts a heavy price on the troubled sleeper.

If you suffered from depression, posttraumatic stress disorder (PTSD), or panic attacks for ten years along with serious sleep difficulties, in most cases you were offered a psychiatric perspective about the sleep disturbances. You probably were treated with therapies or medications focusing on mental health or psychological concerns, and scant attention was directed at specific sleep elements. Rarely would you have been offered a full and accurate explanation for why you were not sleeping.

If your psychiatrist or therapist doesn't put much stock in your sleep problems and doesn't know how to explain them fully or treat them effectively, how much resolve could you muster to take them seriously?

If your past sleep treatment experiences were limited in this way, your view about sleep would be understandable only through the mental framework with which you were incessantly bombarded. Over time, you would learn to interpret sleep through a prism capable of dividing light into fewer and fewer colors until eventually the only color remaining would be a black hole, into which the mental health community often drops sleep problems.

The same scenario plays out for those with insomnia who do not suffer mental health problems but who attribute sleep disturbances to stress. They are told to relax and take stress reduction classes that supposedly eliminate sleep disturbances, which may be true for mild sleep problems. However, this viewpoint lowers the sleep problem to secondary importance while inappropriately elevating the mental thing, in this instance stress, to primary importance.

Whether your issues are stress, mental health symptoms, or mental health disorders, this outdated psychiatric/psychological viewpoint consistently ranks sleep problems beneath mental health factors, which proves to be highly problematic to your health.

Sleep Better, Feel Better

Here's the truth about sleep and mental health, from the mouths of innumerable sleep patients yet unheeded by many primary-care physicians, psychiatrists, psychologists, and therapists:

"You know, if I could just sleep better, I don't think I'd feel so bad."

"I think if I weren't so tired, I would not feel so stressed or depressed."

"If I could get more sleep or better sleep, my anxiety or depression would be easier to deal with."

Many health-care professionals, with all the best intentions, frequently respond to this point of view as follows: "Let's treat your anxiety or depression and see if that helps your sleep."

Technically, your doctor or therapist assigns depression as the primary or major problem, whereas they treat your sleep complaints as secondary or a symptom of this so-called primary problem. Depression *must* be more important than sleep problems. Even if sleeping pills are prescribed, insomnia or poor sleep is viewed as a symptom, not the real problem; yet sleeping pills rarely if ever completely and unequivocally cure anyone's *chronic* sleep problems.

Many people know intuitively a much deeper truth about the relationship between sleep and mental health, and this truth will guide you in your quest for *Sound Sleep*:

"If I could sleep better, I would feel better."

When we permit ourselves to take a fresh and honest look at sleep disturbances in mental health patients, we see that sleep disturbances frequently deserve top billing or at least a costarring role in many more cases than once imagined.

This means that if we treat your sleep problem as if it were a primary or a major health disturbance, instead of waiting to treat it *after* treating your mental health problems, not only might your sleep improve more and faster, but your anxiety, depression, or posttraumatic stress symptoms might decrease more and faster as well. Astonishingly, some sleep disorders patients' mental health problems disappear once sound sleep is achieved night after night.

The reverse is also true. If you do not treat sleep problems, you risk worsening or developing a mental health problem such as depression or PTSD. In some research studies, we are seeing that a persistent or difficult-to-treat case of anxiety, depression, or PTSD may be a hallmark of an underlying, untreated sleep disorder.

Sound Sleep, Sound Mind does not represent a hypothesis, belief, speculation, or dream, but literally reflects genuine knowledge from the growing body of scientific evidence about the relationship between your sleep and your mental heath.

Barrier 5: Brain Strain, Drain, and Pain

Poor sleep quality harms and may ultimately ruin your intellectual capacity. Night after night of bad and broken sleep makes you not as smart as you could be, and sometimes it makes you downright stupid. Sleep restores the workings of your mind by improving your ability to learn new things, consolidate your memory, and enhance your mood, all of which is "brain gain." But poor sleep quality, the opposite of sound sleep, leaves you with brain strain, drain, and pain, our shorthand terms for cognitive impairment.

Cognitive impairment means that your mind is not firing on all cylinders. Memory, concentration, and attention problems are the most common impairments. Most problematic sleepers, including many children and adolescents, suffer from mild, moderate, or severe impairment—"brain strain, drain, or pain." When sleep quality is compromised, deep, restorative, and consolidating sleep is no longer experienced, and the ensuing sleep fragmentation leads to a form of brain damage.

Yes, brain damage!

In particular, your memory, concentration, and attention span are no longer sustained at optimal levels. Some impairments are irreversible, caused by severe sleep fragmentation as well as by drops in oxygen levels during sleep. Some impairments are caused by fatigue and sleepiness, which may be reversible with proper treatment. Much of these impairments are mistaken for aging or for medical or psychiatric diseases. In children and teens, we see lackluster school performances or inattentive behavior and rush to put our kids on medications.

What's most intriguing about brain strain, drain, and pain is that you cannot spot the thing you got!—which, as you are about to learn is why cognitive impairment is the most insidious of all barriers blocking you from sound sleep.

Think about It

The very disease that causes your suffering cripples your ability to see the disease you are suffering from and disables your ability to measure the suffering it causes.

How so? Simply, we all become accustomed to the tools in our own toolbox.

They may be new and sharp when you first use them, but sooner or later they become old and dull. Over time we may not spot these changes because they occur gradually. Even when your tools are not performing well, it is more common to imagine they are working just fine. It's easier, almost natural to see things unchanged instead of questioning one's capacity.

Memory, concentration, and attention are essential tools to make good decisions and proper judgments to live a balanced and prosperous life, which leads naturally to closure on the day. When these mental faculties begin to wear out, you lose some capacity to form solid judgments, make sound decisions, and perceive things accurately, including, as a great example, your capacity to distinguish between the natural effects of aging and the impact of poor sleep quality on your mind. Likewise, you lose the capacity to distinguish between mental health disorders and poor sleep quality's fragmenting impact on your mental health.

As brain strain, drain, and pain set in, they intensify the human tendency to traverse life's highways on cruise control, as if you were sleep-driving your way through life. When you function in this manner, you find yourself heading down the same road, time and again, without paying much attention to the potholes, or worse, to the ditch alongside the road. And because the human mind is inclined to slip into a rut from time to time, once the wheels start spinning, it is difficult to gain traction to pull your mind out of it.

Driving Yourself Nuts

To expand this analogy, consider what happens while stuck in traffic. Because many problematic sleepers suffer fatigue and sleepiness, they react hastily and become frustrated in such encounters. Many drivers ensnarled in traffic complain, vent, or express negative feelings; and there is no law against it unless you perpetrate road rage. However, the value of this strident form of emotional expression is questionable. People who engage in this behavior generate more frustration, tension, and other unpleasant feelings that linger throughout the day. Solid evidence indicates that daily emotional upheavals of this specific type harm your mind, your body, and ultimately your sleep.

You might be the type or know of someone who throws this advice out the driver's side window. For whatever reason, when stuck in traffic, you vent with the best of them or just stew to the boiling point. Remarkably, you engage in these ineffective, self-destructive behaviors for months, years, or decades. No matter how many times you hear suggestions to approach this problem in a new way, you persist in these behaviors not solely because you want to, but because you are literally in a rut in the way you think, feel, and see while ensnarled in traffic jams.

To change this behavior you need attention to watch yourself heading down the wrong path; you need memory to recall what new path you want to take; and you need concentration to sharpen your focus to see the change through until you create a new behavior—say, turning on a golden oldies radio station and singing your way clear of traffic.

No change occurs without effective use of your attention, memory, or concentration.

This example highlights a dilemma for many problematic sleepers. Having lost or damaged the essential tools needed to spot their impairment, they go for years without recognizing how poor sleep compromises their life. Like a needle skipping on a turntable, they are left with a broken-record behavior that prevents them from ever seeing the adverse influences of poor sleep quality.

A fair number of individuals reading these paragraphs categorically deny that it could ever apply to them, and their "thou doth protest too much" mentality all but guarantees that they just cannot spot this behavior in themselves. Although many around them see the devastating effects of bad sleep on their judgment and decision-making, the individual is blind to the problem because he or she has been robbed of the very tools—attention, memory, and concentration—needed to see it.

Barrier 6: Controlling the Control Thing

Of all the barriers, control issues are the most difficult to overcome because sleep is such a mysterious, uncontrollable human behavior, and many of its mysteries remain unsolved. You can willfully choose not to eat or drink for surprisingly long intervals, but you can only voluntarily stop yourself from breathing or sleeping up to a certain point. Just like holding your breath, the longer you try not to sleep, the faster you give in. Most people who seek to stay up all night cannot spend a full twenty-four hours without sleeping; they nod off along the way, if only for a few minutes, no matter how hard they try not to, and even if they do not remember sleeping!

Another mystery involves those who sleep only five or six hours and feel great, while others never feel rested regardless of the number of hours slept.

This mystery—one of the biggest for troubled sleepers—goes unsolved until you appreciate that all sleep is not the same.

Another unsettling mystery surrounds those who labor all day under heavy stress yet still sleep soundly through the night, whereas others perceive a single daytime stressor as a thorn in their sides at night.

No wonder poor sleepers feel that they have little control over sleep. However, this feeling emerges in the wake of a largely forgotten and critical fact: no one has much control over sleep, not even normal sleepers! Sleep is a natural function of mind and body that ought to take care of itself. You get into bed, fall asleep, and remain asleep as long as needed, and that's your bedtime story from start to finish.

If your story is instead one of horror, tragedy, fear, anxiety, depression, frustration, anger, worry, or stress, you are probably trying to control your sleep instead of attempting to control the three things that would solve your sleep problems:

1. poor sleep quality;
2. closure issues;
3. self-defeating sleep habits.

In contrast to any strategies to control your sleep, it is entirely within your grasp to control and correct poor sleep quality, closure issues, and self-defeating sleep habits. You could learn to completely or almost completely control sleep quality within a reasonable time frame—a few weeks to a few months for most troubled sleepers. Control of sleep quality also eliminates many closure issues and learned behaviors.

If that sounds like a fantasy, then let's start daydreaming.

Suppose you wanted advice for a one-week vacation in New Mexico. Because I live there, I could offer suggestions to enhance the quality of your upcoming vacation, and by using selected recommendations as a basis to plan, your trip would be full of experiences of your own choosing. In this process, you probably would have little or no control over the time frame: it might be one week in the summer, which you would have to schedule far in advance. In other words, what you experience during the trip has more impact on the quality of your vacation than the actual time period for the trip.

Our aim is to develop an itinerary to increase your control over the content or the quality of your sleep. To take full advantage of the analogy, keep in mind that most people—but not all—sleep better during vacations, because it's easier to gain closure at the end of the day and to change habits while on a relaxing trip.

Letting Sleep Happen

Our lack of control over sleep does not stop most poor sleepers or chronic insomnia patients from making every effort to control it, despite the fact that sleep-controlling behaviors and habits usually worsen sleep.

Sleeping pills and alcohol are excellent examples of this paradox. Many poor sleepers learn to use these substances to try to control slumber. However, when sedatives (particularly older types of medications) or alcohol are taken every night for months or years to induce or maintain sleep, they further degrade sleep quality. Many people try sedatives but declare the pills do not keep them asleep through the night, just as many who regularly use alcohol near bedtime wake up a lot in the second half of the night.

Choosing a medication or other substance to control sleep almost always produces confused mental pictures about the purpose of sleep; far too much attention is turned toward number of hours slept. Some pills or substances entrench physical dependencies, making it impossible to sleep without them, even though sleep quality is not restored. Eventually your sleep worsens for want of more thorough treatment.

Most troubled sleepers try to control sleep in other ways that also produce unintended consequences. The single most common sleep control behavior is spending more time in bed, hoping to increase sleep hours. In what always turns into a classic, self-defeating, learned behavior, the troubled sleeper thinks he is exerting the maximum control over his sleep by predicting "more time in bed equals more time asleep."

It sounds logical, doesn't it? It might work once in a blue moon. Over time, this control strategy fails because it prevents you from *letting sleep happen*. Worse, once you are frozen to the mattress, you are teaching yourself to stay in bed and *not sleep*, arguably the worst learned sleep behavior you could ever adopt. And that's only the beginning. While not sleeping in bed, aggravating and frustrating feelings emerge that cripple your efforts to achieve mental and emotional closure at day's end. Soon you sleep even fewer hours, despite lying in bed for longer periods. As maddening as lying awake in bed feels, an enormous number of problematic sleepers are mesmerized by this behavior, which rarely breathes new life into their sleep.

Control appeals to most problematic sleepers because most are fairly intelligent, so it seems logical to try to think their way out of their sleep problems. But the more time they spend thinking about sleep, especially while lying awake in bed, a bad habit develops, closure vanishes, sleep quality worsens, hours of sleep shorten, and the old adage is reversed, "More is less."

Most sleep control behaviors backfire because they reflect misguided, largely ineffective, and unsustainable approaches to gaining closure on the day. Every night you could drink beer or wine, take an antihistamine (never combine alcohol with antihistamines), use prescription pills, or lie in bed waiting to fall asleep, believing these strategies are reasonable ways to close out the day. Sooner or later these barriers steer you away from sound sleep, leading you to the same fate as the artist who painted himself into a corner.

SLEEP ON IT
To Thine Own Sleep Be True

QUESTION: Please rate your level of honesty in assessing your own sleep problems:

1. I am very honest with myself about the severity of my sleep problems.
2. I am trying to be honest with myself, but I am also confused about the severity of my sleep problems.
3. I tend to block out my thoughts or feelings about the severity of my sleep problems by keeping busy or using caffeine to get by.
4. Other people tell me I have a sleep problem, but I need convincing.

COMMENT: It is truly remarkable that so many people have a sleep problem, yet so few admit, discuss, or develop meaningful curiosity about it. Most repeat the chorus "I'm just stressed out" or "I'm a light sleeper" and then avoid discussion or investigation. I must confess that these views are not surprising. It took me years to face up to my own sleep problems and recognize how adversely they affected the course of my life and how much they were affecting my mental and physical well-being. Treating them made it possible to write this book.

Sleep problems are health problems, and whenever someone is faced with labeling himself with some ailment, the preferred option is to run the opposite way. This fear of illness commonly occurs with sleep disorders, because they sound like a mental health thing. Sleep carries added baggage, having been tagged with so many disparaging labels: slothfulness, laziness, malingering, no discipline, no ambition, being a slacker, being fragile, being weak, being unfit, and so on. Ironically, severe sleep disorders cause all these problems in a lot of people, so these links are important, but the direction is reversed from what we usually imagine.

We see underachievers all the time in our sleep clinics—individuals who lost their way twenty years back because their exhaustion prevented them from effectively pursuing their life's ambitions. In work, relationships, recreation, social activities, and even spiritual realms, these individuals could not compete or participate at the level they had imagined possible prior to the onset of sleep difficulties. Among children and adolescents, we see many underperforming in school and elsewhere.

Remarkably, we also see many *overachievers* in our sleep clinics, including people who spent years or decades in hyperkinetic lifestyles in which rest and sleep were trivialized or ignored. By keeping busy or using caffeine (usually both) or by ingesting illicit drugs, these problematic sleepers compensated to override embarrassing or uncomfortable feelings about sleep issues, low energy, and mental impairments associated with poor sleep quality.

Strange, isn't it, that the same problem could provoke different people to respond in opposite ways? Yet in both instances, each person has tremendous difficulty in honestly or accurately evaluating the severity of his or her sleep problem.

––––––– PEARL –––––––
What You Don't Know about Your Sleep
Will Wake You Up

This assessment proves difficult for no other reason than you have gone so long without getting the sleep you need, you are no longer capable of honestly knowing what good sleep quality feels like. Even the person who shares your bed is not a particularly reliable eyewitness to your sleep quality because he or she is asleep most of the night and not watching you. A critical step to rapidly advance your progress is to realize that both you and your bedmate may not have skills or tools yet to know for sure what's causing your sleep problems. Honestly admitting this predicament will solve it a lot faster than ignoring or denying it.

4

Sleep in a Bottle

How Did You Start down This Road?

"Sleep from a bottle" seems to make sense. But sleeping pills do not consistently restore sleep quality, let alone solve your sleep problems.

The system might start with once-per-week use. However, if your underlying sleep quality and closure problems are not addressed, "sleep in a bottle" will be used more and more, from a few times per week to nearly every night, after which it becomes in part a learned behavior.

Some ask, "If the system works, why change it?"

Does it really work?

Your natural sleep system is clearly not working, because you learned to depend on a sleep aid instead of your natural sleep physiology that lets sleep happen. Almost invariably, your EEG is still speeding up either at bedtime or during the night, but no one is addressing how to slow down your brain waves with nondrug approaches.

Right now, you do not need to eliminate a "sleep in a bottle" approach. Instead, you need to sort out the real reason or reasons why you adopted this system. Was it due to one or more of the six barriers described in the last chapter, or is it caused by one of the next four barriers common to those who rely on sleeping pills? When you know these answers, it will prove much less daunting to change or discard this incomplete system.

Supervision Needed to Eliminate Sleep Medications

Eliminating sleep medications is often a prudent step to enhance sleep quality. But timing is everything, and SDT does not suggest, recommend, or require that you change your medication in any way without first consulting your prescribing physician. Some troubled sleepers feel that they do better with various types of medications, and it may be painful and counterproductive to consider otherwise. Most others are eager to eliminate sleeping pills. If the material that follows motivates you to change your use of medication, this program strongly recommends that you discuss any changes with your prescribing physician. Changing medication without proper supervision can lead to serious side effects that could land you in a hospital or worse, and changing your use of other substances may cause severe side effects as well.

Barrier 7: Emotional Blocks

Strong emotions lead many troubled sleepers to "sleep in a bottle." Many suffer from emotional turmoil, which they have not learned how to manage in a healthy way. Others may deal with some of their emotions reasonably well, but then they suffer from strong emotional reactions to *not* sleeping. In either case, when you cannot put yourself to sleep or stay asleep naturally, it feels as if you are not performing as you should, which triggers or intensifies emotional reactions. It is tempting, if not rational, to avoid or suppress these reactions and seek quick solutions with prescribed or nonprescribed aids from a local drugstore, health food store, or liquor store.

Unfortunately, like the worried man who drew pictures of himself and thought filing them away each night would "save face," negative feelings related to sleep problems rarely resolve without confronting them. Quick-fix medication approaches often worsen emotional reactions and barriers. In part four you will learn specific techniques to identify and resolve emotional barriers to sound sleep, using methods superior to medications.

Barrier 8: The Unsolved Closure Mystery

Emotional barriers clearly provoke emotional closure problems, which lead many physicians and therapists to see closure strictly as a mental health issue and sleeping pills as the best therapy. However, greater scrutiny of emotional closure often uncovers a different set of feelings that prevent closing out the day—the classic sleep misery triad of sleepiness, tiredness, and fatigue.

You know that dissatisfaction in the day's events leads to unfinished business, and you can imagine how emotional turmoil produces a dissatisfying day. But have you ever stopped to take a closer look at what's really causing the dissatisfaction? In troubled sleepers, chances are extraordinarily high that their low-energy state during the day is causing a lot of the problem. Yet few health-care professionals draw attention to the role played by the sleep misery triad.

Think about it: daytime fatigue, tiredness, and sleepiness impair almost every waking behavior. These pernicious symptoms interfere with the way you think, feel, and see things; they cloud your vision of what's important in life as well as how to extract meaning from daily activities. These sleep symptoms may cause you to eat too much or to eat unhealthy foods; they turn off your sex life; and they turn you into an inefficient and ineffective worker, all of which thwarts your aspirations. At minimum, these symptoms of low energy negate your daily priorities, leaving you with a dampened sense of accomplishment during the day.

How then are you supposed to close out the day . . . when you might feel like you never had much of a day?!

Most mental health patients with sleep complaints are not instructed to look carefully at symptoms of daytime exhaustion as a valid explanation of closure difficulties. Instead, the exhaustion arises from the mental health issue, which supposedly caused all the sleep problems.

By not clarifying this perspective, you would more readily accept a prescription for a sedative or an antidepressant from your provider. Additionally, you might use more over-the-counter sleep aids, drink more alcohol, or use marijuana instead of seeking care from a sleep specialist. Over time, many "sleep in a bottle" systems stop working, and the underlying closure or poor sleep quality problems reemerge in ways that prove deadly for some.

Barrier 9: Losing Sleep over Losing Sleep

Losing sleep over losing sleep is not only a great sleep killer, but also this singularly devastating learned behavior triggers some problematic sleepers to attempt or to commit suicide. Once sleep deteriorates to the point where you expect things to go poorly at night, many sleepers' worries grow beyond the scope or severity of the actual sleep problems. Combine this misery with a failing "sleep in a bottle" method, and insomnia spins out of control. All aspects of sleep worsen:

- taking longer to fall asleep;
- suffering more awakenings or having greater difficulty returning to sleep;
- further decaying sleep quality.

This spiraling produces the ultimate closure problem: the belief that you may never sleep again!

When this worry takes hold, you are guaranteed of losing sleep over losing sleep. As preposterous as the belief seems, the individual who feels this way cannot stop ruminating about not sleeping, and the ruminations prevent the brain from slowing down . . . to sleep. Some individuals' mental and emotional capabilities are so taxed, they reach a breaking point where hospitalization or very potent sedation is required. Psychiatrists and psychologists are skilled in recognizing these crises and the need for urgent treatment. While medication works in the short run to address suicide risks, most people need a new slant to learn how to directly target closure and quality issues without drugs. The proof of this point is that millions of people receive treatments with antidepressants, tranquilizers, and sedatives, yet substantial numbers continue to complain of racing thoughts or anxiety at bedtime as well as insomnia and poor sleep quality.

Many continue losing sleep over losing sleep, yet they assume that the ineffectiveness of the medication is their own fault. Their mental health must be worse than the doctor assumed, so the only answer is more medication. Millions of troubled sleepers have tried a variety of different drugs yet still don't sleep well, still don't erase their racing thoughts, anxieties, and fears, and still don't eliminate mounting worries about losing sleep over losing sleep. Ironically, many medications used separately or in combination can worsen your sleep.

How then can sedatives be so highly touted when so many people who use them still wake in the middle of the night or report minimal improvement in sleep quality after having slept through the night?

Barrier 10: When More Is Really Less

The answer to this paradox is that something else degrades your sleep, which the drug does not address. Either the drug cannot prevent you from waking in the middle of the night, because it doesn't erase the cause of such awakenings, or the drug does not improve sleep quality, because it does not erase the poor sleep quality you suffer from. All of this raises the interesting question of whether sleeping pills or antidepressants give you more sleep, which leads us back to an old answer . . . all sleep is not the same.

Nearly all the older brands of sedatives clearly worsen sleep quality by diminishing delta sleep and promoting stage 2 NREM sleep. Some of the newer agents appear to enhance sleep quality some of the time, but these gains are often less than what you can achieve by uncovering and resolving the mental and physical elements causing your poor sleep quality.

If sedatives do not consistently improve sleep quality or do not improve it to a high level, how do they make you "sleep" more?

The short answer is that sleeping pills may increase clock hours while having minimal or no change in solid hours of sleep. Most sedatives also affect your memory, so you are less likely to remember waking up as much during the night, and therefore it seems you have slept more. Most importantly, it is common knowledge that most sleeping pills and many psychiatric medications speed up brain waves at times and diminish the amount of REM sleep you receive. Yet, these findings are rarely researched for their impact on sleep quality.

All of this raises the following questions: If certain sleeping pills give you more sleep without a marked increase in quality, then are you really getting that much more sleep? Suppose the pill decreased your sleep quality, is it possible you might be getting less sleep?

If someone offered you one ounce of gold or twenty-five ounces of silver, which would you take?

I trust you took the gold, one ounce of which would be worth nearly three times the value of twenty-five ounces of silver. Golden slumbers means deeper sleep; its benefits are more noticeable and valuable than obtaining more sleep of lighter (lesser) quality. As your capacity increases to improve sleep quality, the deepening of your slumber will be so obvious, so pleasurable, and so healthy you'll start dreaming about platinum slumbers, currently worth twice the weight of gold.

Newer Perspectives

These barriers return us to the issue of sleep fragmentation, the speeding up of brain waves that compromises sleep quality. Is fragmentation caused by mental factors, physical factors, or both? Or is fragmentation genetically programmed into your brain waves such that you are cursed with lifelong insomnia?

Chief among the advocates of medication approaches are those who think about sleep through "chemical imbalance perspectives" similar to those who think about antidepressants for depression. In the sleep version, three theories are common:

1. Problematic sleepers, particularly those with insomnia, tend toward excessive arousal activity day and night, which makes them more awake at all times and therefore less likely to sleep.
   - The body shows a higher resting temperature during the day as well as faster, more activated brain waves (fragmented) at night during sleep compared to normal sleepers.
2. Problematic sleepers suffer from unhealthy alterations in neuro-transmitters or neurohormones—important biochemicals that occur naturally in the mind-body—which cause insomnia by preventing sleep onset or consolidated sleep.
   - Specific receptors in the brain, linked to your neurobiochemistry, are targeted to solve sleep problems.
3. Problematic sleepers do not develop these problems of excess arousal activity or imbalances in neurobiochemicals; rather they are inborn, making them susceptible to insomnia their entire lives.
   - The genetic constitution of the troubled sleeper is at fault, and one day, genomic research will cure the problem.

All three of these theories overlap, and each has scientific merit. Sleep Dynamic Therapy (SDT) appreciates the relationships among these theories and faster brain wave activity or sleep fragmentation. However, in our view, these well-conceived and useful paradigms reflect incomplete approaches for treating problematic sleepers. Rarely would these theories *fully* explain the tide of sleeplessness that takes over people's lives. Most importantly, SDT purports that the mind-body has a much greater capacity for change than anticipated by these narrow theories. In sum, we believe the jury needs more evidence before coming to a verdict on this critical issue.

Indeed, many sleep specialists do not believe there is sufficient scientific evidence to support the long-term use of sleeping pills; most do not prescribe long-term sleep solutions with sedatives or antidepressants. In my view, the Food and Drug Administration's recent indication for long-term use of new sedatives was ill-advised. The repercussions of this decision may erect new barriers among patients who seek a more thorough approach to their sleep problems.

At our sleep centers, most patients require extensive evaluations and therapies, including overnight sleep studies, to determine the potential for a "sleep in a bottle" system. In our work, few patients need insomnia medications. We treat hundreds more patients who seek to eliminate their "sleep in a bottle" approach.

Whatever the nature of the sleep aid you use, is it time to look in new directions for help? Rating your sleep quality should help you answer this question.

SLEEP ON IT
Head Bobbers vs. Body Snatchers

QUESTIONS: These next two questions address the final and most powerful influences that push people to use "sleep in a bottle." Your initial responses may prove revealing.

1. When you feel sleepy, where do you feel it?
2. When you feel tired or fatigued, where do you feel it?

COMMENT: Most suspect the questions refer to situations or locations where you feel tired or sleepy, but the real point is about where in your mind and body do you feel these feelings?

Sleepiness is akin to the feeling of drowsiness, the pleasurable sensation that occurs prior to falling asleep. You want to lie down when sleepy. Fatigue or tiredness may or may not be pleasurable; it's something you can feel in various situations: after extended physical activity or exercise; when your energy level is low but you are not sleepy or desiring sleep; or when your mood is bored or depressed. You often want to sit down and rest when you're tired or fatigued.

So the "where" of sleepiness is in your head or mind, whereas fatigue and tiredness are something you notice more in your body. When you are sleepy, it is difficult to hold up your head; it may literally bob up and down as you try to stay awake. Your eyelids become heavy; it is difficult to keep them open. Your mind drifts and loses focus, seeking the natural and presumably healthy escape of sleep, given the right circumstances. Sleepy feelings should be pleasant, especially if circumstances permit sleep, but they can generate frustration or anxiety, even pain if driving a car or meeting a deadline.

Fatigue or tiredness is felt more in the body than in the head or mind. Your muscles might be sore or achy. Your body doesn't have the energy to do anything in particular, almost as if the energy had been snatched or stolen from you. If you force yourself to do something while tired, it may generate painful or frustrating feelings in your body.

Many people with sleep disorders blur the distinctions between these feelings and lump them together, which is especially problematic for someone with insomnia, because the insomniac will try to fall asleep when tired but not sleepy. Worse, some insomniacs are confused by the previous sentence, asking, "Is there really such a precise difference between feeling sleepy or tired?" Because they have lost the ability to make these distinctions, they resort to the "sleep in a bottle" approach.

In the treatment sections you will learn that if you do not sense the experience of sleepiness primarily in your mind and fatigue and tiredness primarily in your body, then you will need to explore these perceptions to ensure success in the program. The treatment sections will show you how to use these distinctions to solve your sleep problems.

Can you detect the difference between sleepiness and fatigue? Can you rate your sleepiness vs. your fatigue and tiredness currently experienced in daily life? Can you see how you would be tempted to use sleeping pills if you did not feel sleepy at bedtime or during the night?

––––––– PEARL –––––––
Your Natural Sleepiness Is the Most Powerful Sleeping "Pill"

When you measure these feelings, please note:

- Tiredness describes a recent feeling during a particular day or after a particular event.

- Fatigue is more commonly used to describe chronic tiredness.
- Sleepiness is distinct from both conditions.

These distinctions are critical to your success with SDT. Understand this point, and all your treatment steps will go more smoothly, **because virtually every human possesses a natural ability to generate and experience sleepiness or drowsiness just prior to falling asleep**.

This *Wave of Sleepiness* is your ultimate ticket to *Sound Sleep*.

5

Solving Your Sleep Quality Puzzle

Quality Control

Now is the time to face *Poor Sleep Quality . . . the monster itself.*

With the Sleep Misery Index you rated a series of symptoms often connected to poor sleep quality. Now let's get personal and link these symptoms to how you actually feel and function in your daily life, so we gain the most accurate measure of the problem. As you work on these steps, do not hesitate to reread sections on any barriers if they block your path.

To simplify, you only need to focus on one concept in this final self-assessment: energy!

In each of the following three scenarios, notice how your perceptions of high or low energy reveal much about your sleep problems:

1. How refreshing or unrefreshing do you find your sleep upon awakening in the morning?
2. Is your morning routine filled with get-up-and-go?
3. How much sleepiness, tiredness, or fatigue do you notice in the afternoon or evening?

The Lucky Ones

Normal sleepers' responses to these questions prove enlightening because they:

- find sleep very refreshing;
- feel great upon awakening in the morning;
- might spring out of bed singing "Oh, What a Beautiful Mornin'" and rarely start the day with caffeine;
- have little or no daytime sleepiness, tiredness, or fatigue, and find themselves mentally sharp much of the time;
- rarely use caffeine in the afternoon or evening;
- do not make lifestyle choices to cover up or distract themselves from sleepiness, tiredness, or fatigue;
- have relatively high and constant energy most of the time to meet the needs and demands of their lifestyles, including a rich capacity to be as physically active as they desire;
- suffer no closure problems or self-defeating learned behaviors at day's end to interfere with their capacity to sleep soundly all through the night.

These individuals do not pay attention to how many hours of sleep they obtain each night, and regardless of the number, their clock hours and solid hours of sleep are nearly identical. Because they are blessed with consistently outstanding sleep quality, the number of sleep hours needed each night is remarkably consistent. Yet if they miss an occasional hour of sleep, it does not cause a problem.

So do normal sleepers' patterns depress you, or can you imagine the great things you have to look forward to?

The Unlucky Ones

Most poor sleepers or those with insomnia describe their sleep as unrefreshing, both mentally and physically. "Unrefreshing" means you do not feel refreshed when you awaken in the morning. This term is exceedingly important, because most people with unrefreshing sleep demonstrate clear-cut sleep fragmentation when tested at most sleep labs. Thus "unrefreshing sleep" is a reliable indicator of a sleep disorder, which often includes unsuspected physical components such as breathing or movement disorders.

Spotting the unrefreshing nature of your sleep indicates you are not recharging your batteries night after night. This single insight advances your analysis of your sleep problems, because you know the impact of the sleep disturbance yourself, instead of needing someone else to point out the problem. Unfortunately, many poor sleepers who honestly admit they suffer from sleep problems still declare their sleep refreshing, perhaps because some nights are better than others. Sleep Dynamic Therapy (SDT) assumes your sleep might be partially refreshing, but wouldn't that make it partially unrefreshing, too?

Some poor sleepers declare "My sleep is fine, I just need more of it." Usually their attention and anxiety are stuck on number of hours slept each night, although some truly need more hours. Among patients seeking treatment for sleep complaints, the "sleep fine, more sleep needed" expression almost always heralds a sleep quality problem, too.

If you discern your sleep as unrefreshing, you are ahead in the game. If you believe your sleep is refreshing, you may be correct, as each situation is unique. Chances are high, though, you are using "refreshing" in a way that does not accurately describe your sleep. As we continue, try to add more precision to your use of the terms "refreshing" and "unrefreshing," so you better appreciate how all sleep is not the same.

The Morning Hangover

If sleep supposedly restores you each night, you should feel great in the morning, right? Or consider the reverse: if sleep supposedly restores you, would it make any sense to feel any or all of the following in the morning or soon thereafter?

- desire to remain in bed longer;
- needing to hit the snooze button several times before getting up;
- desire to sleep more;
- feeling of not enough sleep;
- feelings of sleepiness, tiredness, or fatigue;
- need for or the habit of using caffeine or other stimulants to start the day;
- believing you are not a morning person;
- cranky or irritable attitude;
- inability to think clearly or concentrate on something;
- overall uneasy, tense or otherwise unpleasant feeling about starting the day.

If you suffer from insomnia, you might ask, "Couldn't these beliefs, attitudes, and feelings all be caused by insufficient sleep?" For insomnia patients, the less sleep you get, the more you suffer; but to reiterate, the problem of *Poor Sleep Quality* caused the reduced number of hours in the first place.

Suppose you usually sleep five or six hours but one night you slept eight hours. If you can recall such an experience, then answer these questions:

1. Why were you able to sleep longer on that particular night?
2. Why did you feel better in the morning after that particular night?
3. Why can't you repeat this cycle with the same good results night after night?

Most insomnia patients respond "I don't know" to the first or third question and "I slept longer" to the second. SDT offers more meaningful and useful answers to the same three questions:

1. Better sleep quality let you sleep longer.
2. Better sleep quality made you feel better.
3. You're not getting better sleep quality night after night.

You did not improve sleep quality by sleeping more hours; you slept longer hours because your sleep quality improved for some reason on that night. Your morning hangover symptoms would diminish after such a night because you attained much greater sleep quality.

Connecting the *Zzzots*

Now that you understand the nature of unrefreshing sleep and the morning hangover, the last step assesses your energy level and its impact on functioning throughout your day. Sleepiness, tiredness, or fatigue are the most obvious drains on your energy during the day, but now you are ready to answer more global questions that expand on the Sleep Misery Index:

- If sleep restores physical and mental energy, how do you connect any particular night of sleep with your energy level the next day?
- Can you naturally link fatigue or a lack of concentration during the day with a troubled night of sleep?
- When you are worn down or tired or stressed out, could you be getting older, or could you be getting bad sleep?
- How do you make this last distinction when you are unaware of the science showing poor sleep makes us older faster?
- If your memory declines, when do you blame aging, or when do you blame poor sleep quality?
- When you learn that poor sleep causes serious memory problems, which are reversible with sleep treatments, would memory loss still be explained as a natural part of aging?

- When depressed, how do you know if it's biological depression or the depressive symptoms caused by a sleep disorder, or both?
- When anxious, irritable, tense, or stressed out, do you think that these symptoms reflect anxiety or stress disorders, or that they are caused by years of invisible sleep fragmentation, a condition often mistaken for a mental health problem?
- How might you determine whether your doctor or therapist is confusing your sleep condition with a mental health disorder?

Most troubled sleepers have thought about these questions, but almost always in the back of their minds. When they try to discuss these ideas with physicians, they are usually not greeted with enthusiasm.

More *Zzzots*

The next list meets the same fate. These items are so common in day-to-day life, everyone assumes they are normal behaviors—"being human"—instead of a sign of *Poor Sleep Quality*:

- undesirable or excessive periods of daydreaming;
- spacing out;
- losing focus;
- forgetting or misplacing things;
- dropping things, especially small objects;
- mishandling things;
- bumping into things;
- feeling off balance;
- making simple or silly mistakes;
- other mental lapses.

Notice how all these occurrences arise from a lack of mental or physical concentration, as if mind and body become uncoordinated. Unquestionably these behaviors are excellent indicators of underlying sleep quality problems.

For some people, dangerous microsleeps—very brief episodes of actual sleep—invade and temporarily wipe out awareness or concentration, which can lead to motor vehicle crashes or other serious accidents. Most people do not imagine that these mishaps indicate a problem, even after suffering a car crash or a close call behind the wheel!

Sleep fragmentation (aka *Poor Sleep Quality*) during the night contributes to all this daytime dysfunction. Most poor sleepers do not connect these dots, so they compensate instead.

Compensatory Actions

The verb "compensate" means "to make up for a lack of something else." A compensation does not fix a problem; it sidesteps it to get by. Crutches are great compensators for a broken leg, but when the leg heals, you want to walk on your own without compensating aids.

How do you compensate for a lowered energy state? The following responses are common:

- You recognize your daytime fatigue and sleepiness, then treat it with appropriately timed naps, caffeine, other stimulants, and precise restrictions on what you can do in your life.
- You ignore fatigue and sleepiness yet somehow plow ahead with willpower, caffeine, adrenaline rushes, or perhaps anxiety.
- You ignore *or* recognize fatigue and sleepiness, then adopt an extreme, if-you're-not-moving-you're-dead lifestyle in which you rarely sit down or remain motionless or quiet for more than five minutes (knowing you might doze off if you did).
- You throw in the towel, knowing something is wrong with your energy level; yet you try to plug the leak, so you alternate between resignation and depression or frustration and anger.
- You crawl through life, never knowing you were saddled with an extra, nearly invisible burden every day.

Despite the variation in responses, notice that most people sidestep whether sleepiness, tiredness, or fatigue have definable causes. Most look at energy drains as if compensating were the only solution.

The Drive to Thrive

Why are there such variable responses among troubled sleepers?

Ambition often seems to determine how compensating lifestyles take root.

People with relatively low ambition, potentially induced by severe sleep problems, often set their sights lower in life. They may not perceive any impact of sleep problems on their ambitions and may not recognize they have developed low ambitions. They just live a life with few aspirations.

In contrast, some with higher ambitions who also suffer severe sleep problems push forward for some time in at least a few (but rarely all) realms of life. These people make gains with the use of willpower; caffeine; adrenaline rushes; or anxious, hyperkinetic energy. Their constant struggle with low energy produces a gross lack of balance. When a person must push all the time to achieve any goals, a price is paid along the way, because too much energy is spent in one place and not enough is left over for other realms. A person might be ambitious at work and have a major letdown in family or social life. Such a person drops onto the couch in the evening with only enough energy to watch television. Or such people put most of their energy into their family or social life and muddle their way through work.

You have observed many people living out their lives with high or low ambitions, but you may not have connected their behavior to sleep problems. Obviously, cultural, societal, and personal influences push people in numerous directions, but sleep problems contribute to their lifestyles as well.

SDT appreciates that it's normal to find ingenious, imaginative, and creative ways to compensate and get by or to move forward in life when energy reserves are too low. You must find the energy somewhere, or give up. For those who move forward, it is remarkably human for some poor sleepers to set high ambitions, then develop unique blends of caffeine, willpower, adrenaline rushes, and anxiety to forge ahead.

Solving Your Personal Energy Crisis

Would fixing your sleep problems solve your energy issues?

For those with high ambitions, could you imagine maintaining these ambitions without caffeine, adrenaline rushes, or anxiety and without needing every ounce of willpower on any given day? For those with low ambitions, could you imagine the possibility of a life with more energy and higher aspirations? In either case, can you imagine the distinct possibility of going through the day in an entirely new and more relaxed mode because the energy you need is always there, always available, and always ready for use in your daily life?

For just a moment, can you picture:

- waking up feeling refreshed and starting off the day with a full head of steam?
- how it would feel at midmorning *not* to be yawning, needing coffee, or needing a break?
- the *absence* of a postlunch energy dip?
- *not* needing to fight off fatigue or sleepiness during an uninspiring afternoon meeting?

- gaining enough energy after dinner to forgo the couch or boobtube and instead play with your kids, work on a hobby, or enjoy socializing with friends whenever you choose?
- possessing all the vibrant energy you need to enjoy your jam-packed days until the end of each day without having to *push* yourself the whole way there?

These rewards are just the physical ones. What about the mental and emotional rewards?

- Can you imagine a clearer mind in the morning and for most of the day?
- Can you imagine better concentration and a more reliable memory?
- Would newfound energy help you cope with the stressors in your life?
- Would daily frustrations and irritations be more easily overcome with abundant energy at your disposal?
- With energy reserves to spare, would your temper be so quick?
- Could you picture a life in which anxious and depressive feelings are more easily overcome because your energy level provides the necessary drive to do something about these disabling emotions?

Sounds exciting, doesn't it?

When your sleep quality is restored, can you predict the impact on your daytime fatigue and sleepiness, your mental and physical health, and on the *rest* of your life?

SLEEP ON IT
Rating Your Sleep Quality

QUESTION: Now is the time to make an educated guess about your sleep quality. Select one of the following to complete this sentence: "For most nights, on average, I experience . . ."

- Very good sleep quality.
- Good sleep quality.
- Fair sleep quality.
- Poor sleep quality.
- Very poor sleep quality.

COMMENT: Comparing how you feel after a good night versus a poor night of sleep is another way to assess sleep quality. You could experience one night of great sleep quality and observe how you felt after sleeping so well. Then you could experience one night of poor sleep and see how you felt. Afterward, compare the two nights.

This method sounds logical, but do you see the flaw? For a valid comparison, you must experience good sleep quality firsthand, but if you were a poor sleeper, how would you know when your sleep achieved high quality?

For those who selected fair sleep quality or worse, you have either known for some time or you have begun to realize that your sleep quality is a critical part of your sleep disturbance. If your assessment is accurate, the following could be true:

- A person with very poor sleep quality probably has a very severe sleep quality problem.
- One with poor sleep quality might have moderate to severe sleep quality problems.
- One with fair sleep quality probably has a mild to moderate sleep quality problem.

Spelling out these possibilities aids you over time because your perceptions of what it means to sleep well change as your sleep quality improves.

Some may have selected good or very good sleep quality, which reminds me of the story of the poor man who lived in a hut with a three-legged stove. The man kept dreaming about buried treasure under a bridge hundreds of miles to the south. When he traveled to the bridge, he hesitated in his search for the treasure, which soon provoked a guard, who asked him what he was doing. When the poor man told him the dream, the guard laughed and said, "Why, if I believed every dream I had, I would have walked hundreds of miles to a little town in the north where I would find a poor man who lived in a hut with a three-legged stove, and I would dig for buried treasure under his stove." The poor man made his way home, uncovered the buried treasure that had been hiding there all along, and lived happily ever after.

——— PEARL ———
Emergency Sleep Treatment Focuses on Sleep Quality

Some troubled sleepers persist in linking sleep quality to their sleep quantity, maintaining they always feel better when they get eight hours compared to six hours. However, you would be surprised at how many people with insomnia or poor sleep report the opposite. They feel worse when they sleep longer, so they adopt the strategy of sleeping shorter. A huge proportion of people with poor sleep—millions in the United States alone—adopt this shorter-sleep approach consciously or as a learned adaptation over time.

This shorter-sleep method treats their sleep disturbances up to a point, because your worst sleep quality may coincide with the last hour of sleep. Cutting off the worst sleep quality by awakening earlier may improve sleep. Also, cutting down sleep time tends to decrease fragmentation and increase consolidation. And because cutting down sleep also tends to make you feel sleepier at bedtime the next night, this strategy overcomes closure problems and self-defeating learned behaviors at the end of the day.

By treating the problem this way for years, these troubled sleepers forgot how the process evolved. They no longer think of themselves as having sleep difficulties. In both the short and the long term, the less-is-more approach has value and benefit for some individuals. However, SDT does not recommend sleeping less as a curative treatment, because this method does not fully treat the underlying sleep quality problem. It does not resolve all sleep fragmentation or resolve all closure issues or self-defeating learned behaviors. Ultimately, although shorter sleep may serve as an excellent stopgap measure, it quickly inflicts significant sleep deprivation on most who attempt it.

6

Countdown to Sound Sleep

If It's Broken, Fix It

We are into the final countdown to the formal treatment steps of your personal Sleep Dynamic Therapy (SDT) program. You were asked to evaluate new ideas and approaches to your sleep problems, and I thank you for your patience. I also purposely avoided many typical questions you have probably seen, heard, or read about elsewhere, such as:

- What time do you go to bed?
- How long does it take you to fall asleep?
- How many times do you awaken during the night?
- What time do you wake up?
- And, of course, how many hours of sleep do you get each night?

These questions may prove crucial, particularly to someone who has rigid schedule demands that interfere or conflict with efforts to sleep. Shift workers might need to pay more attention to them. Even so, these questions pale in comparison to what you are learning about sleep quality, closure problems, and self-defeating, learned behaviors, because these three critical elements ultimately determine:

- the time you go to bed;
- the time it takes to fall asleep;
- the number of times you awaken at night;

- the time you wake up in the morning;
- the total time you spend sleeping.

You may have been exposed to a health-care professional or even a sleep specialist with limited training or experience in managing insomnia problems, who focused on these items while showing less interest in your sleep quality. They may have suggested a number of sleep hygiene instructions to address these items. "Sleep hygiene" refers to a set of behavioral suggestions about your sleep habits, patterns, and behaviors, as in the following list.

SLEEP HYGIENE INSTRUCTIONS

Attempt to:

Go to bed only when you feel sleepy. Establish and maintain regular bed and wakeup times.

Find the amount of sleep you need to feel consistently refreshed.

Create a comforting, quiet, clean, and dark environment for sleeping. Your bed and bedroom temperature should be comfortable.

Establish a regular pattern of relaxing behaviors 10 to 60 minutes before bedtime.

Use the bedroom and bed only for sleeping and making love.*

Exercise regularly.*

Start your mornings with some sunshine.

If possible, do not:

Nap during the day or evening.

Eat heavy meals or drink large amounts of liquid before bedtime.

Dwell on intense thoughts or feelings before bedtime.

Lie awake in bed for long periods of time.

Allow your sleep to be disturbed by your phone, pets, or family.

Use alcohol, caffeine, or nicotine; all of these worsen sleep.

---

*Sex and exercise have different influences on individuals. Let your personal experience guide you in adjusting these activities as they affect your sleep.

Source: ©Krakow & Smith 1993

These instructions prove useful, depending on how they are presented, how much depth you appreciate lying beneath their surface, and how consistently you apply them. Some sleep hygiene instructions are remarkably powerful and actually repair portions of broken sleep. For example, if you drink caffeine near bedtime, you might worsen closure problems and increase sleep fragmentation at night. Changing this behavior reduces closure issues and improves sleep consolidation.

Sleep Hygiene Pros and Cons

The larger question about sleep hygiene is whether you can follow the instruction (for example, no caffeine past 2:00 P.M.) to change the behavior. There may be practical and productive reasons for drinking caffeine later in the day or evening (driving home safely). Or your desire to change this behavior may require too much effort when first tackling sleep problems.

SDT allows that sleep hygiene instructions are useful, but we find they work better and have lasting effects if you first repair your broken sleep with stronger therapies. Once sleep quality problems start resolving and most closure barriers are removed, sleep hygiene instructions are easier to apply. After initial treatment successes, you'll discover that sleep hygiene makes it easier to overcome self-defeating behaviors.

Sleep hygiene work is paradoxical, and the best example of a paradox is the instruction for regular exercise. Many troubled sleepers do not exercise because they are tired and cannot muster the energy to maintain a routine. If exercise were attempted, a tired or sleepy person commonly feels exhausted afterward, and many are prone to injury and accidents during exercise.

Might exercise help you sleep? Sure, a good twenty- or thirty-minute walk may help, but don't be surprised if you feel more fatigued afterward, and take care to prevent yourself from tripping over curbs or twisting your ankle. The wiser approach is to fix sleep quality first, gain a substantial increase in energy, and then discover the joy of exercising and the wide-ranging rewards it brings. This approach is safer and sustainable.

Among severe insomniacs, trying to fix sleep problems first with sleep hygiene is akin to asking a diabetic to coax his pancreas to make more insulin. The first three items on the sleep hygiene list epitomize this problem.

Establish and maintain a regular bedtime and wake-up time every day. How could you establish this routine if your biggest problem were falling asleep at the start of the night? The instruction makes no sense until you overcome the major closure problem. Using a set wake-up time might help, but if you were still concerned with the number of hours slept, this instruction might lead to shorter sleep.

Go to bed only when you feel sleepy. All right, but what if you suffer from severe insomnia and never feel sleepy before bedtime? This problem indicates you have difficulty distinguishing feelings of sleepiness from feelings of tiredness or fatigue. You have to solve this problem first to use the instruction.

Find the amount of sleep you need to feel consistently refreshed. Once determined, sleep that number of hours. For some, this instruction begs the question. The rule assumes your sleep must already be refreshing, so just figure out how many hours of supposedly refreshing sleep you need. But most readers are now clear that their sleep is not refreshing, so there is no sensible response to the instruction.

Many sleep specialists praise sleep hygiene instructions. However, if you lose focus on the major objective to resolve sleep quality problems, sleep hygiene instructions prove to be like Band-Aids used to pull together a much deeper and wider wound that really requires sutures.

Please consider the sleep hygiene instructions briefly. If you find an item that pertains specifically to your problems and feel comfortable trying it, then do so. Never select an isolated sleep hygiene instruction that frustrates or annoys you. There's not enough to be gained by sleep hygiene right now if it causes emotional distress. Many have already tried these steps and found them difficult or useless, usually because they were not linked to solving underlying sleep quality problems.

Sleep hygiene instructions appear here because these instructions are not a major focus of treatment in a SDT program.

Aim Higher and Higher

SDT provides many innovative, nondrug techniques to solve poor sleep quality, closure issues, and self-defeating sleep habits. The methods were developed from many sources of knowledge from years past, primarily from the works of the great psychiatrists in the late 1800s and early 1900s, innovative psychologists from the 1940s through the 1960s, and pioneering sleep researchers from the 1950s through the 1980s. Our research team has added steps that we have published in the scientific literature as well as some techniques from our clinical and research experiences. SDT has attempted to integrate all these ideas into one comprehensive program.

As you start treatment, keep this single point in mind: *you may not appreciate how much improvement you can possibly gain until you gain all the improvement possible.* Once you notice you are sleeping a little bit better, don't make the mistake of thinking this improvement is "all the better" you get. *Sound Sleep* offers a quantum leap forward in your life, after which you would never want to return to the ways you used to sleep and suffer.

Don't wish upon a star; aim for the stars.

The Sleep Cavalry

My goal is not to raise false hopes, because each person has a different response to the program. But if you might achieve an 80 percent or a 100 percent level of sound sleep, I want to ensure that you attain this level and not a lower one, which you might believe is all the success you can achieve.

Which brings us to the main character of our story, for you, *my dear sleeper*, are about to enter into a realm the likes of which you might never have dreamed possible.

Some of you have known that your sleep was broken or damaged in various ways for a long time. Many of you have known something was not quite right with your sleep without really understanding what that meant or how to take advantage of this insight. And then there are those who have given up along the way, resigned in so many ways to a life of insomnia or poor sleep.

If you have felt frustrated, angry, or hopeless, you are not alone, and I promise you there is a way out. So listen carefully:

Do you hear that bugle sounding in the distance? That's not reveille cracking your dawn, rousing you from your broken sleep, to start you on another foot-dragging, exhausting, and overwhelming day. It is the sleep cavalry, and we have the knowledge, the tools, the energy, the vision, and above all the duty to rescue you from the sleep misery that afflicts your life.

With the knowledge gained in this SDT program, you will learn to sleep well and soundly through the night, night after night, and finally get the sleep you really need. Change is simply waiting for you to reach out and grasp it.

For some, sleep will become supernormal, which might be a little scary, because not only would you sleep through the night, but you also would gain a huge increase in your daily energy. Truly, a new sharpness and clarity in thinking can prove such a shock to your system, you might suffer "a bout of temporary sanity," in which your capacity to make judgments and decisions is so improved from what it was, you feel compelled to question the changes.

You may be unsettled by the extraordinarily relaxing impact of healthy slumber on your mind and body. As healthy slumber produces one of the most reliable sources of human energy, you may not need to muster any extra energy from artificial means, such as living a hyperkinetic lifestyle or being dependent on caffeine. You soon discover that you can relax knowing your energy savings account receives nightly and substantial deposits from the sandman; and you might be astonished by the "compound interest" you receive from these sound sleep investments.

Make no mistake about it: if you can improve your sleep quality, you will improve your ability to function in just about everything you do each day, and you will enhance your mental health and physical health as well. The results often feel like you have changed your life.

There really is a great deal of truth to the old adage "Sleep on it." The secret is your sleep must be of a very high quality to reap these benefits. Peace of mind the old-fashioned way is genuinely achievable by taking advantage of this twenty-first-century vision of healthy slumber.

Sound Sleep and a *Sound Mind* await you.

SLEEP ON IT
Miles to Go before I Sleep

QUESTIONS: What is the basis of your motivation or your motivation problems? Are you ready to move forward? Or are you nervous about what might lie ahead? Many factors influence your desire to gain good sleep, and it's worth knowing how you rate your motivation as you start the program:

- I am motivated and enthusiastic about solving my sleep problems.
- I am motivated, but I still have a lot of questions about the whole thing.
- I have mixed feelings about treating my sleep problems.
- My motivation is not very strong right now.
- I want to fix my sleep problems to please or satisfy someone else in my life.

COMMENT: In whatever place you find yourself, the most important thing is to be honest about it. If your motivation is high, that's great, but if it's low, being honest about it is the fastest and most reliable way to find new ways to up your motivation.

One way or another, if you have miles to go before you sleep, then please start walking now. Within twenty minutes or less, you'll pass the first milepost. A few miles later, you'll see *Sound Sleep* just ahead. The journey may take a few weeks or months or maybe longer for some, but it could be the journey of a lifetime.

———— PEARL ————

A Commitment to Sound Sleep Lasts a Lifetime

Don't sleep on it; just take that next step.

PART TWO

LAY YOUR MIND TO REST

Sleep Thoughts to Let You Sleep through the Night

Slow Down and Sleep

Let's distill everything you have learned into one idea: the mind, the body, and the brain waves often "move" too fast to sleep or to sleep well. Sleep Dynamic Therapy (SDT) teaches you to slow things down to achieve *Sound Sleep* by showing you how to enhance sleep quality, close out the day, and unlearn self-defeating, learned behaviors. Although we work in small steps, each step, including all the "Little Big Steps" in parts two through five, can produce big results. Some steps require several days or a week or more of attention to properly digest. Rereading sections, especially "Little Big Steps," proves crucial to your comfort and success. The key is learning to fly SOLO.

Going SOLO

Use the SOLO technique to pace yourself through the program. Consider this technique as a basic yet critical tool, placed on top of all other tools in your sleep recovery toolbox. When you start a new step, first pull out this tool. The SOLO acronym means:

S = *Stop doing* (for a few seconds to a few minutes).

O = *Observe* yourself; know your mind.

L = *Let* yourself *be*; just breathe.

O = *Observe* yourself; know your body.

When you apply the SOLO technique, you step back from or move beyond ordinary things in life. For just a few seconds or a minute, you change your perspective to observe yourself with a fresh outlook. Each time you use the SOLO technique, you increase your chances of successfully applying the treatment steps, because you do so with greater conviction and because you monitor your changes with greater candor.

The Human Brain's Mastery of the SOLO Technique

To master your SOLO skills, you must appreciate the way the human brain works. Every human brain has a rich capacity to think, feel, and image, and most behaviors arise from these three actions. Before you eat, you *think* about food, *feel* hungry for food, or *imagine* a picture of food in your mind's eye. All three actions might be engaged before, during, or after eating, whether you live to eat or eat to live.

These Thoughts, Feelings, and Images represent your *TFI System*, and your SOLO skills enable you to watch the flow of TFIs as they course through mind and body.

Three specific things occur during healthy TFI flow:

1. You let many TFIs enter your awareness.
2. You know how to pay attention to the most valuable or relevant information from any cluster of TFIs, depending on desires, needs, and circumstances.
3. You know how to let the rest of the TFIs "come and go."

In the chapters ahead you'll learn how your SOLO skills and *TFI System* naturally complement each other and how they can lead the way in your efforts to overcome psychological and physiological causes of sleep problems.

7

Day Is Done

The Sleep Not That Binds

Sleep Dynamic Therapy (SDT) starts with something so bold, it seems contrary to anything you ever thought, believed, or heard about insomnia or poor sleep. You cannot go to sleep at bedtime, cannot go back to sleep in the middle of the night, or cannot obtain high-quality sleep because:

You really do not want to be asleep! Seriously!

How could SDT propose such a provocative idea? "You might not want to be asleep" smacks of blame, as if you control your sleep.

But blame is not behind this theory, because we repeatedly discussed:

- Sleepers do not control their sleep.
- Sleep is something that occurs naturally.
- Sleep is something you must let happen.

Why then such a bold theory? You really do not want to be asleep!

For example, when you develop the seemingly useful but actually useless learned behavior of looking at a clock in the middle of the night and counting the hours of lost sleep or the hours of desperately hoped-for sleep, not only are you not sleeping, you instead are engaged in the wakeful, learned behavior of time monitoring and calculating. As much as you might argue you want to sleep, in the heat of the battle you are engaged in an active behavior that can only be attempted while awake.

Does it really seem possible that a person could be asleep and awake at the same time? Consider the wisdom of arguably the greatest Yogi of the twentieth century: "How can you think and hit at the same time?" The great catcher of the New York Yankees, Yogi Berra, may not have been talking about sleep, but the analogy holds: you cannot engage in behaviors or habits of wakefulness and expect yourself to sleep.

Consider closure problems. Suppose you had a bad day at work or a conflictual day with your kids. If you bring unfinished business to bed, it's no surprise that you would not fall asleep or stay asleep, right? Part of you wants to finish the business, and that part of you cannot close out the day. Sleep is not welcomed into what should be the sanctity of your bedroom, because some part of you wants to be awake, *not asleep*, to take care of business.

Consider sleep quality problems. When it is fragmented, your mind-body possesses some awareness of broken sleep. Why then would you want to sleep? If sleep is not expected to provide a pleasurable, satisfying, relaxing, restful, useful, or positive experience, but instead feels unpleasant, annoying, restless, dissatisfying, or negative, would you look forward to falling asleep or staying asleep?

More often than you would expect. You really do not want to be asleep!

Common Denominator

In nearly all circumstances that prevent or break up sleep, SDT teaches: You really do not want to be asleep because *Your Day Is Not Done!* As simplistic as this idea sounds, it speaks volumes of truth and provides tons of information. After lights out, you never hear "Taps":

Day is done, sun is gone,
From the lake, from the hill, from the sky.
All is well, safely rest.
God is nigh.

You rarely hear "Taps" because your day is prevented from coming to a close by myriad elements, some of which are obvious and some so deeply hidden within your mind-body it takes weeks or longer to see their destructive influence.

At bedtime, if you could learn to embrace the feeling in your mind, body, and spirit that your day is done, then in most instances you would fall asleep and stay asleep most of the night. Curiously, your sleep quality also improves somewhat.

When you invest in the *Day Is Done* idea, you take back the night by falling asleep or returning to sleep faster than you would with sleeping pills, because once you embrace the idea, a moment later . . . an enormous *Wave of Sleepiness* is sure to follow.

This feeling of sleepiness is so intense because it is a natural, evolutionary part of human physiology, built into your mind-body to force you to fall asleep or return you to sleep. You would never confuse this *Wave* with feelings of tiredness or fatigue. All through the night, it laps at your shoreline, continuously soothing you to sleep.

For many problematic sleepers, day is *not* done makes sense; but they may not accept the idea of "you really do not want to be asleep." Sounds perplexing, doesn't it?

Many troubled sleepers rebel against and dismiss this not-wanting-to-sleep concept. Yet your mind-body and brain waves often have a specific agenda, ready and waiting when you get into bed or when you wake at night, and the first item on that agenda is . . . to stay awake!

Once you rigorously scrutinize this agenda, you can connect this undesirable desire to stay awake to many of your problems with sleep quality, closure, and learned behaviors. With these connections you can figure out what it takes to believe, truly believe, at the end of the day—in both mind and body—that your *Day Is Done*.

Making this change sounds like a big step, but let's turn it into a little big step.

Little Big Step 1: One Night at a Time

After dinner tonight or a few hours before bedtime, please make a short list of things that prevent you from feeling like your day is done. Make a list of unfinished business regarding future events and troubling thoughts or feelings about past events that interfere with sleep.

Remember to start with your SOLO technique:

S = *Stop doing* (for a few seconds to a few minutes).

O = *Observe* yourself; know your mind.

L = *Let* yourself *be*; just breathe.

O = *Observe* yourself; know your body.

Without the SOLO technique, your mind is distracted, and it takes longer to make a list. The SOLO technique sharpens your focus by giving you immediate access to your best powers of concentration, which makes future steps and exercises go faster and smoother.

If you are not sure what to include on your list, here are examples: finances; work; kids; marriage; relationships; home; neighborhood; your state, country, or the planet. And don't forget concerns about your sleep. As you develop your list, be precise but not elaborate. Just use scratch paper, nothing formal; you can toss it later.

If you have a specific concern about work or your kids, spell it out with a few more phrases so you can honestly state in words what's nagging at or troubling you. Keep it brief and to the point; no short stories or novels are needed.

This step is not a technique for writing away your worries, which requires a different set of instructions. Unless you receive specific training and essential feedback on that technique, you could worsen your worries by trying to "write them away the wrong way."

Once you complete the list, review it while pondering this question: "Can I solve any of these problems tonight before I go to sleep?" The SOLO technique proves crucial to your efforts to answer this question honestly, especially when your day has been stressful and you find it difficult to unwind.

Since most of your concerns developed over the course of days, weeks, or months if not years, in most instances the obvious answer is "I cannot solve these problems before I sleep."

If you can solve a particular problem, please do so, but as most concerns require more time, resources, and energy to solve in the future, you now want to ask yourself whether you believe that your *Day Is Done* or at least coming to a close soon.

The most important part of this instruction, right now, is whether you recognize the nature of this granddaddy of all closure issues—that is, can you see how unfinished business, even unfinished sleep business—losing sleep over losing sleep—places you in the undesirable position of not really wanting to sleep because your day is not done?

Can you see how the items on your list might be leaking into your evening hours, causing a stain on your brain that prevents sleep?

Day Is Done in Action

The list you made prepares you for the next instruction, close to bedtime. Sit quietly where you will not be interrupted. Spend no more than five minutes on this step, including a one-minute SOLO exercise to start. Try to convince yourself that the day is really done. Don't work too hard in your efforts, but try the following approaches:

- Persuade yourself logically with appropriate thoughts.
- Persuade yourself emotionally with good feelings.
- Persuade yourself visually with nice images in your mind's eye.

(More is to follow in the next Sleep on It section, on how to use the *TFI System* with the aid of your SOLO skills.)

During this reflection, if a simple idea comes into your head to do something, such as jotting down a reminder for tomorrow, then do so to persuade yourself that the day is done.

You are not trying to trick or deceive yourself into believing that your day is done. You could not do so if you tried! Do your best to move your mind-body in a new direction to feel like and ultimately believe that your day is done.

Then go to bed.

If you discover you cannot achieve a *Day Is Done* feeling tonight or are not sure how to achieve it, you really achieved more than you know.

How so? Because now you see a clearer picture of what needs to be worked on to solve your sleep problems. Now you know you must learn to experience the *Day Is Done* before you sleep.

If you had some success, try to recapture this feeling at any time you find yourself in bed *not* sleeping. When things enter your brain or body, move back to the sensation that the day is done. Reciting "Taps" or another song, poem, or prayer works wonders sometimes.

You are not likely to fool yourself about this feeling, because when your *Day Is Done*, you would almost always feel the pleasurable *Wave of Sleepiness* carrying you to sleep.

If your day really is not done, you might feel tired or fatigued instead, but you wouldn't feel sleepy. If this point is confusing, return immediately to the Sleep on It section at the end of chapter 4 to revisit the distinctions among sleepiness, tiredness, and fatigue. For severe insomniacs, these distinctions are critical to success, because ultimately you want to avoid the bedroom when not sleepy.

In the meantime, if you are frustrated in bed, consider getting out of bed for just a few minutes or more and ask yourself again, "Tonight, can I find a way to finish my unfinished business?" If you persuade yourself that the business can be left unfinished, or that past troubles can be dealt with tomorrow, perhaps it will reassure you that your day is done.

If you have trouble with this first step, fear not. Most troubled sleepers cannot readily appreciate the depth of the *Day Is Done* concept or easily believe it is possible to achieve. Usually something is missing from their perspective or in their personal skills that prevents them from successfully closing out the day.

The missing factor is almost always a question of balance.

Introduction to the "Sleep on It" Treatment Program

Sleep on It sections now consist of two components. The first part includes questions and comments on skills training to develop your *TFI System*; the second offers specific Pearls to treat sleep problems as fast as possible. Your SOLO technique aids you in developing your *TFI System* and in trying out these therapeutic steps.

SLEEP ON IT
Balancing Acts

QUESTION: TFIs (Thoughts, Feelings, Images) enter your awareness to offer ideas and information to review. As your review unfolds, you gain access to as much of your thoughts, feelings, and images as needed to function well, while letting go of information likely to prove meaningless, unhelpful, or harmful. As people mature, they apply some form of the SOLO technique to their review, which helps balance TFIs efficiently. The SOLO technique quickly spots what really needs to be focused on and aids you in letting the other stuff come and go.

Many poor sleepers develop habits and behaviors thwarting the natural balance in their *TFI System*. They learn to fear this review and mistakenly imagine it would overwhelm them. Over time, they develop more rigid, controlling systems that block out valuable information that could offer a fuller life and better sleep. Making matters worse, sleep fragmentation destroys the natural capacity to balance things, because you feel too tired or sleepy to review your TFIs. Without balance, it is nearly impossible to unlearn learned behaviors, find closure on the day, and enhance sleep qual-ity. *Sound Sleep* may elude you until you begin balancing your *TFI System*. It is no surprise that this process takes time, but not a lot of time each day!

Take a SOLO minute to ask yourself "How does my brain use the *TFI System*?" Then rank these three brain activities according to which ones you rely on most and which ones least.

COMMENT: Most people with sleep problems suffer a TFI imbalance of too much time thinking, promoting faster brain waves. Many poor sleepers have a relatively higher level of intelligence, making them too smart for their own good as far as sleep is concerned. They try to think their way out of their sleep problems, but too much thinking itself promotes learned behaviors and closure problems that sustain sleep disturbances for years or decades.

Why do so many problematic sleepers develop a style of excessive thinking if it doesn't help sleep problems and might worsen them? The short answer is that they are uncomfortable with or fearful of their feelings as well as the pictures in their mind's eye, so they think instead. The long answer takes time to discover. The greater your curiosity about this ques-tion, the faster you arrive at its answer.

When poor sleepers try to observe how they think, feel, and picture things in the mind's eye, an immediate concern is whether they comprehend the precise meanings of these brain activities. The many forms of thinking include words, self-talk, or chatter without beginning or end as you go through the day. Because much of your waking life involves working, problem-solving, making decisions, planning, and reacting, you need to think a lot to accomplish your goals. Thinking feels like it occurs in your head, brain, or mind.

Feelings are sensed in the body, although you must develop a great awareness in your mind, too. Feelings involve a broad spectrum starting with barely noticeable things such as putting on your clothes or brushing your teeth and proceeding to intense sensations such as bumping your knee against a chair, the joy of watching your child at a dance recital, or the anx-iety of an upcoming discussion with your boss. Use "feelings" to mean all sensations felt in your body, but use "emotions" to mean a group of feelings linked to positive and negative things. Pain and pleasure are in a special class not typically called emotions, but are linked to emotional experiences. Depending on how you were taught to recognize feelings and emotions, they will be imperceptible, or overwhelmingly on display, or somewhere in between.

Images form pictures in your mind's eye during waking or sleeping situations. You may use imagery regularly if you were encouraged as a child or learned it as an adult. You may be oblivious to imagery if your mind's eye went undeveloped. A person who notices things—sees things—in the environment tends to have a healthy imagery system, whereas those who overlook visual cues or miss the pictures in front of their eyes tend to have weaker imagery systems.

——— PEARL ———
A Balanced Mind Is the Foundation
of Sound Sleep

To understand your use of these three brain processes—your *TFI System*—do not measure the percentage of time in which you engage in these activities. That's impossible. Focus on the concept of balance, which means developing the capacity to experience all TFI elements in a healthy flow, moderated by an unpressured come-and-go attitude.

If you think too much, observe this lack of balance. For feelings and images, the most common imbalance is their absence, although some people experience them in excess, which also speeds up the brain. Please use the SOLO technique for a few minutes each day, observing these three brain activities. Sense how your mind-body operates and its state of balance.

If you were napping during your Childhood 101 class, when the operating manual for this ingenious system was discussed, then spotting TFI imbalances proves tricky. When your mind races along above the speed limit, it's obvious you think too much. Usually you do not realize these racing thoughts emerge from a void created by ignoring the images in your mind's eye or by failing to sense feelings in your body. Imbalances due to missing elements are the most difficult to detect, because it's more challenging to spot something that's not there.

8

Are You in the Wrong Time Zone?

Changing Your Mind

"How many lightbulbs does it take to change a psychiatrist?"

"Just enough to see the light."

Your personal capacity for change determines how rapidly you achieve *Sound Sleep*. Your capacity to change is tied directly to your use of the SOLO tool to see the light (observe yourself) and then balance your *TFI System*. Although the SOLO skill is one of the most powerful tools for change, many troubled sleepers need more guidance in changing behaviors. To steer you, SDT incorporates three common change approaches through the remainder of the program:

- Behavioral: offers instructions to change, then you follow it.
- Cognitive-behavioral: adds more explanation to the instruction, clarifying connections between the way you think and the behavior you want to change.
- Psychodynamic: looks deeper at these connections and helps you gain insights about the ways your thoughts, emotions, and images affect the behavior you are trying to change.

What's most revealing about the change process is whether you can follow instructions to see the change through. Can you learn to move away from the self-defeating *Day Is Not Done* barrier at night and toward your *Day Is Done* solution at bedtime? Can you welcome the *Wave of Sleepiness* into your mind-body and let it carry you to sleep and keep you asleep as long as needed?

In these next three chapters you'll work on these objectives through each of these systems of change. We'll begin with something that takes no time at all.

Dogging It

Have you ever heard of Pavlov's dogs?

They were taught to salivate as if meat were in front of them when actually they were responding to the sound of a bell. Pavlov showed meat to the dogs and naturally they salivated; then in the next experiment, while showing them meat, he also rang a bell, and of course they salivated again. In the last experiment, he just rang the bell *without* any meat, yet they still salivated. By teaching the dogs to react to the bell *only*, Pavlov produced a learned behavior.

A learned behavior or "conditioning" indicates an association or a connection between two things, such that one thing triggers the other, as if a reflex. You notice early in life that a stove emits high heat that burns, so you move in the opposite direction if you experience intense heat unexpectedly. When suddenly exposed to a fire, you wouldn't say "I am experiencing strong feelings of a heat sensation, so I think I'll move away." You would see the fire and feel the heat, and without thinking in words, jump back or move as needed to relieve the heat sensation.

Many people learn this behavior by suffering a small burn, and once learned, this behavior becomes entrenched in your mind-body, over which it seems you have little control. You engage in many learned behaviors throughout the day; many are positive, but there are many opportunities to develop behaviors to make life miserable. You can learn to overeat and suffer from obesity; to overuse alcohol and suffer from alcoholism; and to scream and yell at your kids and diminish the pleasures of family life.

The worst of these learned behaviors is learning to believe that you cannot change your behavior, which, of course, might cause you to do just that—not change it!

Wasting Time

Time monitoring and calculating are two of the most common and troublesome learned behaviors plaguing problematic sleepers. As many as 90 percent or more of insomnia patients fuel their sleeplessness by losing sleep over losing sleep through obsessions about time at bedtime or during the night. Time may heal all wounds, but it will not heal your sleep. Nothing more clearly demonstrates that your day is not done than wasting time monitoring or calculating when you should be sleeping.

For most troubled sleepers, time is an enemy and never an ally. When you bet the odds lying in bed awake, stuck to the mattress, holding out for a chance to fall asleep or back to sleep, you are playing a long shot that rarely pays off. This view seems strange, because it sounds so logical to spend more time in bed to get more sleep. And this reasoning pushes your mind down a path toward calculation after calculation as you attempt to figure out how much time or sleep is left in the night, if you were to fall back asleep in thirty minutes, an hour, or two hours, and so on.

Time becomes your master and you its slave with respect to your bedroom and sleep habits. We are all slaves to time because we are mortal, but time has no place in the bedroom; and sharing your bed with time eventually leads your sleep to serve your bedroom with divorce papers. Yet sleep and your natural *Wave of Sleepiness* are the first to skip out. The result is chronic insomnia.

Little Big Step 2: Beat the Clock

The powerful connection between sleep and time was developed earlier in discussions about sleep quantity. Now it's time to eliminate this self-defeating behavior. If you have already altered this behavior, that's great. Use the following material to learn new ways to overcome other learned behaviors that disrupt your sleep.

A simple one-night experiment helps break the sleep-time connection:

- Turn the clock in your bedroom to face the wall so you can never see what time it is during the night (you can still use the alarm).
- If awake at any point in the night, **make absolutely no attempt to**:
  - determine what time it might be;
  - calculate how many hours of sleep you have obtained;
  - figure out how many hours of sleep you may still get;
  - figure out how long it will take to fall asleep or back to sleep.
- In sum, completely eliminate behaviors at bedtime or at night that have anything to do with time or calculations.

Now go SOLO for one minute and consider these questions:

- What did you immediately think about these instructions?
- How did these instructions make you feel?
- Did you picture being in your bed without access to a timepiece?

Before turning the clock around, bear in mind that many with moderate to severe insomnia do not embrace these behavioral instructions. Frequently, insomniacs cannot easily give up time monitoring and calculations and therefore require more than behavioral techniques.

Can you see this change through?

Time Doesn't Pay

When you monitor time in bed, you are creating a learned behavior that prevents sleep. You desire sleep, but you engage in a behavior that alerts you and speeds up your brain waves. Once alert, spying the clock or figuring time points gives you a sense of control over your lack of sleep, but this useless feeling of control blocks your natural Wave of Sleepiness from washing over your mind-body to carry you to sleep.

In virtually all circumstances when you monitor time or make calculations about sleep quantity while lying awake in bed, you are teaching your mind-body that the bedroom is not a place to sleep. The bed and the bedroom are where you watch clocks and worry about time. As with many learned habits, you connected two behaviors: checking the time and not sleeping, which fuel sleeplessness.

To paraphrase Yogi's question, "How can you think and sleep at the same time?"

The more obsessed you become with time—mulling over the time it takes to fall asleep, the number of times you wake up, the number of hours of sleep you will or will not get, and the time you must wake up in the morning—the more time infects your sleep so your day is never done. This infection spreads through the mind-body, speeds up the brain, and soon destroys your sleep quality, intensifies closure problems, and feels like an irreversible learned behavior.

Time Obsessions

Mild insomniacs engaged in time monitoring cure their insomnia just by turning the clock to face the wall. However, success occurs only when—with the clock gone—they also stop their calculations about time and about how much sleep they're losing, getting, or needing.

More is at stake for those with severe sleeplessness because they suffer from anxiety, depression, posttraumatic stress, or other emotional strife. This emotional turmoil plays havoc with their efforts to balance their *TFI System,* and it distorts their time perceptions, making it more difficult to give up time monitoring.

At minimum, troubled sleepers must accept that clock-watching activates the mind-body. You have too many associations with time that have no relationship to sleep. When you ask what time it is or check the time, you are doing or planning something. You need time and a schedule to eat, work, play, run errands, keep appointments, talk to friends, enjoy family life, and smell the flowers, and you need to fit sleep in somewhere, too.

In the daytime, it is useful to look at the clock and figure schedules. You would neither want nor need your day to be done, during the day, because your day is not over.

The same mind-set of keeping pace with daily life does not work with sleep. It worsens sleep quality by activating your body to imagine you control sleep in the same way you control your schedule. Yet no amount of conscious effort of this sort ever controls sleep. Monitoring time ruins your slumber because it stimulates you to think and ruminate about your sleep as if it fit into an empty space on your calendar. Sleep rebels in the face of time pressure, and your *Wave of Sleepiness* dissolves, leaving you with tired feelings that don't herald slumber.

This issue is not a simple matter of not looking at the clock while in bed. You need to give up other ruminations about time during the night as well.

Time Out

Suppose you turned the clock to face the wall to prevent time-monitoring behavior if awakened at night. Then suppose you can't get back to sleep after awakening. Would the absence of a clock prevent you from monitoring time?

Absolutely not! Without a clock, nothing prevents you from noticing the degree of darkness outside, listening for the sounds of birds, observing the position of the moon or the intensity of moonlight, hearing the frequency and pattern of traffic outside, or looking for any other clue to drive yourself nuts. If none of these behaviors provides information about time, you can always guess the time based on how you slept before you woke up, whether you woke up from a bad dream or a noise, or whether you awakened feeling drained and tired or strangely refreshed and enlivened.

If you want to do the math on how much sleep might be yours before dawn, you can always find a way to guess or watch your environment to gather information to fuel your calculations, ruminations, and worries. Once you go down this path, the most accurate description of your behavior, whether or not it resonates with you, is: you really do *not* want to be asleep; you want to be awake to monitor time.

Until you break this habit, it remains extremely difficult to experience your day as done, gain a full sleep recovery, and reap the rewards of *Sound Sleep*.

Most troubled sleepers have difficulty giving up the clock with basic behavioral instructions, so we'll explore cognitive-behavioral and psychodynamic elements in the next two chapters to aid your quest to break the time barrier.

SLEEP ON IT
Erasing Racing Thoughts

QUESTION: Most poor sleepers recognize that racing thoughts or worried thinking (ruminations) afflict them at bedtime or in the middle of the night; they point to this excess mental activity as a primary cause of sleeplessness.

Take a SOLO moment to reflect on your experiences with racing thoughts or ruminations at bedtime or during the night, including worries about time, then answer this question: "Why is it so difficult to turn off my mind when I go to sleep or after an awakening interrupts my sleep?"

Draw up a short list of reasons (in your mind) that explains this excessive brain activity. Give yourself another SOLO moment to reflect on your answers before reading the comment.

COMMENT: The short answer to explain racing thoughts and ruminations is that your wheels are already spinning most of the day, so why stop at night? During the day, you may notice an activity in your mind resembling racing thoughts, ruminations, or time worries, but because you remain active in so many ways, you don't perceive this thinking style as problematic or as an imbalance in your *TFI System*.

For certain situations, thinking and doing work well together, creating a seemingly ordered or structured life based on words in your head and actions in your body. An ordered life generates a sense of control, which adds to the appeal of thinking and doing.

Sleep is the opposite of this waking experience; you are not doing, ordering, or controlling. When you try to sleep, virtually all doing stops; when you fall asleep, you are vulnerable and not in control; and when you dream, rarely would you call this imaginative experience orderly.

But if you hop into bed with a waking mind-set of thinking and doing, you suddenly find yourself holding a sleeping bag full of racing thoughts and ruminations that do not easily come and go. Excessive thinking—a key to feeling in control while awake—isn't useful at bedtime. Once this groove wears into your brain, not only do you keep thinking and thinking in bed (speeding up brain waves), but also you may not know how to turn off the flow of ideas when seeking slumber.

The long answer to the problem of racing thoughts and ruminations, then, has everything to do with how you learned to think, feel, and picture things during the day, not just at night. Excessive thinking rarely emerges magically when you try to sleep. Ruminations are ever present, lurking beneath your radar during waking hours. At bedtime your radar spots these racing thoughts, which visibly and annoyingly interfere with your sleep quest. Racing thoughts are mostly your antidote to feelings and images that seem less controllable, because excessive thinking keeps these elements at bay. However, the more you ignore your feelings or images, the more imbalanced (excessive) your thinking becomes, which speeds up the brain and prevents sleep. Most troubled sleepers do not know what to make of this point.

Consider a wheel, which possesses three parts—a hub, spokes, and a rim. We can assume that correctly linking all three parts produces the roundest, most balanced, and most useful wheel. Many problematic sleepers do not correctly link all three parts of the *TFI System*, but instead suffer one of life's greatest illusions by creating a false sense of order and control through excessive thinking.

For now, please consider the potential for hidden pressures to build when you stuff feelings or images. This pressure fuels racing thoughts and ruminations. Occasionally you glimpse the fuel (emotions) fanning the flames; more often you perceive only the flames (racing thoughts).

When you function this way for a long time, you develop a belief that these two essential elements of the *TFI System*—feelings and images—should be avoided as much as possible. You perceive emotions and the pictures in your mind's eye as troublemakers that herald the coming of unpleasant and undesirable feelings such as anxiety or fear. You believe that feelings and images cannot come and go. This fear of fear may prove to be your greatest obstacle to balancing.

Understanding the precise details of this imbalance and creating a new balanced system take time, effort, and perseverance, but your progress leapfrogs ahead when you let your healthy curiosity accurately observe the current state of your *TFI System*.

———— P E A R L ————
Set Your Bedroom Clock to All Sleep, All the Time

The fastest way to grasp these concepts is to apply them to your everyday life. For most problematic sleepers, time monitoring provides an excellent target. If you are a troubled sleeper who happens to not watch the clock, substitute something else from your daily life (perhaps obsessing or worrying about bills or your diet) as you use the next steps.

First, spend a day or so observing what goes on in your mind-body when you look at a clock (or when you think about finances or diet). You might find it easier to look at a clock during the daytime, but inevitably, if you cannot give up time monitoring in bed, you must notice what you think and feel while looking at the clock at night.

Use the SOLO technique, then explore what you think about before, during, and after spying the clock. During waking hours, you would be planning something or determining whether you are on schedule. Pay close attention to how your thinking sparks certain emotions, pleasant or unpleasant, depending on what you connect to time and your pursuits on the day.

At night, what emotions do you connect to time monitoring? If you are not sure, start your exploration by first listening to your thoughts when you spy the clock. Most troubled sleepers plunge headfirst into mathematical gyrations to calculate all possible scenarios remaining in the night. With careful observation, notice how your calculating thoughts trigger unpleasant emotions that start with frustration and anxiety and that can unleash a torrent of more unpleasant and intense emotions, including anger or fear, all of which block your natural *Wave of Sleepiness*.

When you observe with great precision, you are likely to see that the first feelings you notice in yourself actually trigger more interest, obsession, or thinking about time, which raises a chicken-and-egg question: "Which came first, the thoughts or the feelings?"

A great reward awaits those who spot the connections between their thoughts and feelings when monitoring time at night, because awareness of these connections makes it much easier to break the time barrier.

9

Breaking the Time Barrier

Just in Time

If your time bomb is still ticking in your bedroom, let's try cognitive-behavioral therapy (CBT), which provides more material to change your perspective on time. By making a change in your thinking (cognitive), you may find it easier to change your behavior (behavioral).

If you tried to turn the clock around yet struggled to avoid monitoring time or crunching sleep numbers, you know that mental anguish and emotional strife usually hitch a ride along this dreary path, fueling closure problems and corrupting your *Day Is Done* efforts. Perhaps you imagined that too much strife would arise with this change. Frustration and anxiety, if not the whole gamut of unpleasant emotions, may erupt when you give up time monitoring.

Time monitoring and calculating, then, are psychologically or emotionally driven processes. And because you know that psychological and emotional factors affect the entire mind-body, you would not be surprised that time monitoring speeds up your brain waves and damages your sleep quality in a physical way as well. Making matters much worse, once you eventually fall asleep, brain waves do not necessarily slow down. Your mind-body may carry this burden into your sleep.

Time marches on . . . and on . . . stamping out sleep from your brain through more sleep fragmentation. Instead of descending into deeper, consolidated, restorative stages of slumber, you cycle between being asleep and being awake, spending too much time in stage 1 NREM, even though you have limited awareness of this pattern. This harmful cycle could be programmed into the mind-body by watching the clock.

The physical effects caused by time monitoring and crunching sleep numbers cannot be easily measured, but the impact is not small, given that nearly all troubled sleepers who give up time-monitoring behaviors report clear-cut improvements in sleep quality or the feeling of deeper sleep.

Are you still sure you want to "Rock-a-Bye Baby around the Clock"?

Sleep-Wake Confusion

Making matters unbelievably worse, sleep fragmentation caused by time monitoring contributes to one of the worst misperceptions in the life of a poor sleeper. Time monitoring could distort your capacity to distinguish between being asleep or awake. This distortion seems implausible, but for those with moderate to severe sleeplessness, confusion arises about whether they have nodded off at times. In severe cases, insomnia patients cycle between sleep and wakefulness at such fast rates, they feel like they didn't sleep at all.

You might sleep for one minute, then arouse or awaken slightly for fifteen seconds, then continue this exhausting cycling for hours on end. Some sleep for longer periods, but sleep is so light—often stuck in stage 1 NREM—the same confusion arises. This sleep-wake confusion corrupts your *Day Is Done* experience and your efforts to recruit the *Wave of Sleepiness*. If you feel like you didn't sleep, then you feel like your *Day Was Never Done*! It's as if you wanted to jog over to the market but instead found yourself unintentionally running in place . . . for hours! There is no useful slumber gained with this cycling, and it often leads to mere ripples of sleepiness instead of the *Wave* at bedtime.

Time monitoring and crunching the sleep numbers physically injure your sleep quality. Each time you spy the clock, you program the physiology of your mind-body to stay awake while you attempt to sleep. You might as well put out a fire with gasoline!

Little Big Step 3: Just Enough Time for Sleep

These new insights into how time monitoring worsens your sleep raise four questions:

1. Has this information encouraged you to make a change in behavior?
2. Do you now accept that time-monitoring behaviors are incompatible with sleep?
3. Do you really want to be asleep, or do you want to watch the clock?
4. If you used a different example such as obsessing about your weight or your finances, can you see how this ruminating type of thinking prevents you from sleeping?

For some, the next steps may be less about immediate changes and more about learning to analyze your reactions to the instructions. Remember, use the SOLO technique to notice any thoughts, feelings, emotions, or images that arise:

1. Start with the *Day Is Done* exercise early in the night or before bedtime.
2. After step 1, spend an extra minute pondering this question: "If time waits for no man or woman, why should I wait for time?"
3. Next, before getting into bed, spot anything coming up about time. Are you worried about:
   - what time you are going to bed?
   - how much time it will take you to fall asleep?
   - waking up and losing sleep time?
   - not getting enough total sleep time?
4. Observe reactions and emotions triggered by thinking about time, and then use your new insights about the uselessness of time monitoring to let go of these worries.
5. Now, to the best of your ability, in your mind, declare clearly and sincerely the following sentiment: "I don't really have time for this, because it's time to sleep."
6. Then see if you can catch the *Wave of Sleepiness*.

Time Passages

You now know that watching the clock and engaging in the mental math not only produce emotional anguish, but also these behaviors physically fragment your sleep quality and radically impair your chances for obtaining deeper, refreshing, and life-enhancing slumber.

This information spurs some troubled sleepers to make necessary changes. Yet even in the face of this important physical connection, poor sleepers feel reluctant to give up their awareness of time as they grasp for sleep. None should be surprised, though, for we only need to consider another behavior in which individuals cannot easily stop, namely smoking. A smoker hears repeatedly about lung damage, cancer, emphysema, asthma, allergies, and even the unhealthy influences of smoke on friends, family, and coworkers, but this information may factor only a bit into their ultimate decision to quit smoking. This fact-checking approach may have little impact because it ignores the major reasons why the smoker continues smoking: the individual enjoys something about it, feels benefit or comfort from it, or gains a sense of control while doing it.

So, too, poor sleepers who monitor the clock or crunch sleep numbers like to do it or may feel as if they benefit or receive comfort or control from time monitoring, even though it developed as a learned behavior. As odd as it sounds, they are more comfortable when their day is not done, which means there must be some benefit when you really do *not* want to be asleep.

If we wish to explore this benefit, we need to dig deeper for a cause, which brings us to the psychodynamic model. When you hear "psychodynamic model," you might be the type who immediately conjures up anxiety about a deep, dark psychotherapeutic process sure to uncover a miserable, nasty secret that has been hidden for years.

Perhaps, but the first thing that might more usefully come to mind about "psychodynamics" is the proverbial tale of Nasrudin when he lost his key and scoured the grounds outside his home in search of it. When a neighbor offered to help, the search continued unabated until his friend inquired, "Where did you lose the key?" Nasrudin calmly replied, "Inside my house." To which his exasperated friend asked, "So why are we searching out here?" "Because," exclaimed Nasrudin, "there is more light."

SLEEP ON IT
Controlling Your Control Issues

QUESTIONS: The most likely benefit gained from time monitoring is a greater sense of control, but the real question is "Control over what?" An unhealthy desire for control is most often a desire to manage an unpleasant or unwanted emotion, such as anxiety, worry, discomfort, frustration, a sense of insecurity, or outright fear. When a poor sleeper spies the clock and thinks over and over again about time issues during the night, she is often covering up an uncomfortable feeling, such as:

- anger or frustration about reduced sleep quantity;

- anxiety or stress about the next day's affairs;
- fear or panic about the hazards of not sleeping.

The major flaw here is using "thoughts" to solve an "emotion" problem, whereas, the entire *TFI System* is best suited to address feelings and emotional concerns. Although you may not fully understand this technical point yet, recall that a balanced *TFI System* permits a healthy flow of thoughts, feelings, and images. Frequently TFIs are just visiting and have no motive to take up residence in the mind-body. As a child, you understood that TFIs came and went. But when poor sleepers forget or no longer accept this principle, they gradually corrupt their systems; they learn to block a natural flow of TFIs because they expect to be overwhelmed or hurt by their feelings or the images in the mind's eye. Thinking too much, especially if you are smart—as are so many troubled sleepers—is the best way to control or block feelings and images.

In psychodynamics, time monitoring is the mind's attempt at distraction, because your mental gymnastics reflect an intense and loud form of verbal chatter in your head. Time chatter diverts attention from undesirable feelings and images . . . for a while.

To understand this point most clearly, consider these two questions: When you obsess about time issues, what feelings or emotions are you trying to control? Have you considered managing these feelings or emotions in new ways other than by time monitoring? Or ask these questions about other obsessive thinking patterns.

COMMENT: Many troubled sleepers are perplexed by these questions because they do not analyze time monitoring or other learned behaviors in light of feelings and emotions. At night, many have vague feelings of tension and discomfort or emotions of anxiety and frustration, but rarely do they see how clock-watching intensifies emotions or diverts attention away from one's feelings.

If you cannot identify your emotions with precision, it will be difficult to see their influences on your sleep. Some individuals never received normal cues on healthy emotional development and suffer from severe emotional and sleep problems, leading to irrational fears about giving up the clock. They have been stung so badly losing sleep over losing sleep that fear grips mind and body when trying to solve any sleep issue. Some come dangerously close to a mental breakdown, and time-control obsessions hasten this breakdown.

Troubled sleepers must consider the possibility that when feelings or emotions push you to use time-control, you not only lose the battle against time but also the war to conquer sleep problems. In the heat of the night, you must appreciate that if your objective were to ignore your feelings or emotions or the images in your mind's eye, then technically this means just one thing:

It's more important for you not to sleep, because you would rather ruminate about time instead of spending any time with what you are feeling or picturing in your mind's eye.

How certain is this point?

Pretty certain! Your need to avoid feelings and images can only mean you are willing to let your thoughts race, which you know makes sleep impossible. Racing thoughts arise because you mute your feeling button. As emotions are turned off, the volume of mental chatter turns up, and your mind-body cannot lead you to sleep. Truly, you really do not want to be asleep, which explains how too much thinking is a sure bet to keep you wide awake and keep your *TFI System* off balance.

Sleep Dynamic Therapy teaches that the fastest way to gain control over your sleep is to give up control of it! The first step in unlearning any of your sleep-controlling behaviors requires you to dust off your built-in emotion detector to identify unpleasant or unwanted feelings. You must learn to recognize these hidden TFI elements that force you to use time-control strategies.

─────── PEARL ───────
Stop Spending Your Emotions
Winding Up the Clock

Before you identify and attend to feelings or emotions triggered or covered up by time-monitoring behaviors, you must assess your comfort level in working with them. You may proceed on your own or with a therapist. This first exercise teaches a basic truth about emotions and does not require psychotherapy. Remember, apply the SOLO technique.

The next time you feel frustration, give yourself five or ten seconds to identify the frustration and notice how it feels in your body. Do not mistake this pearl for psychobabble. This step may take days or weeks to master. Many prone to overdosing on thinking need longer to learn to identify and feel their emotions. So ask yourself:

- What does frustration feel like?
- Where are you feeling it in your body?
- Does the feeling change, or move to different parts of your body?

If you are not ready to work on a feeling such as frustration, notice simpler feelings before tackling intense emotions. Feeling your hands hold this book is a feeling. Notice whether you hold it with a little or a lot of tension. Many but not all troubled sleepers find they have too much tension in their hands. Those are two feelings: the feel of the paper or book jacket on your skin, and the tension in your hands holding it.

Most importantly, can you distinguish between feeling a feeling and thinking about one?

Spend only a couple of minutes each day identifying specific feelings and emotions and measuring your capacity to feel these feelings and emotions. See if you can complete this exercise without too much self-talk dampening the experience.

More in-depth instructions are in the chapters ahead. Three reminders for now:

1. Use the SOLO technique to start any practice with feelings or emotions.
2. Feelings will come and go, which is part of the experience you want to master.
3. Never forget: time is not of the essence!

The entire process goes more smoothly as soon as you recognize that the emotions you are trying to avoid are the same feelings that push you to think too much.

10

The Sands of Time

Life and Death

Life is very short. So much of our lives pass by in no time at all that at some point in time we realize there may not be enough time left to fulfill our life's ambitions. The dimension of time has great meaning to all of us, whether or not we are clock-watchers. During key episodes in our lives, new awareness of the Big Clock sharpens and enriches our appreciation of what we do in the world and increases our motivation to find meaning.

September 11, 2001, is a remarkable example of this phenomenon, in which millions of people around the globe collectively raised these meaningful questions: "What's important in my life? How do I spend more time engaged in these important things?" When you accept and appreciate the shortness of life in a positive and uplifting manner, it leads to a great sense of renewal, which redirects your energies and passions toward the achievement of your ambitions and your heart's desires. It also makes it easier to gain spiritual closure at night, if that proves important to you.

Remarkably, when a transforming process occurs in the hearts and minds of some traumatized people, it produces a spiritual healing. It were as if highly stressful experiences serve as a wake-up call, much like Michael J. Fox referring to himself in his book, *Lucky Man*, after developing Parkinson's disease. The overwhelming experience leads to a special awareness of self not perceived previously. In kind, the old adage "adversity introduces us to ourselves" was among the first messages from President George W.

Bush after September 11. When we learn about ourselves in this way, time pressures unexpectedly ease.

Regrettably, this positive, uplifting, if not spiritual, new awareness of one's life, does not always occur following intense events. Many survivors have an opposite reaction in which life seems to get shorter without the renewal and redirection of energy, and without the promise and hope that new meaning will be realized. Instead of managing time more effectively, these individuals feel added time pressures and might become daytime clock-watchers. Though one eye scans the digital display of a wristwatch, another eye or the mind's eye become more invested in the Big Clock and how much time might be left in a lifetime.

Spiritual Misery

Spiritual closure problems at the end of the day push the *Wave of Sleepiness* far out to sea.

This unenlightening version of adversity is seen among certain trauma survivors, including many with unresolved sleep disorders. Their disabling fatigue and sleepiness drain their energy and sap the will right out of their minds and bodies. Their productivity drops off for almost everything in their lives, even routine, daily chores and activities. As daily functioning declines, more time pressures build, because these survivors cannot keep pace. At bedtime, many trauma survivors surely feel like the day is never done, and their sleep misery worsens their frustration, anxiety, or fear. While these emotions originated from trauma, now they are compounded by exhaustion that cripples their coping abilities to get through the day.

How could such people find closure when they are perpetually vexed by these questions:

- If it's another rotten night of sleep, where does the energy come from to get through the next day?
- If sleep does not occur naturally, how ugly is a trade-off between pills or substances needed to sleep and a hangover that follows?
- What guarantee is there of getting a minimum amount of sleep?
- Will six hours of sleep get the job done the next day . . . five hours . . . how about three hours . . . what number will satisfy tomorrow?
- How am I supposed to cope when sleep seems so very far away?
- What the devil am I supposed to do if sleep never comes?

If you have ever gone down this path, it is crucial to realize that it is natural, almost predictable that you would wrap up your fears and frustrations into obsessions with clock-watching. Yet if you remain unaware of these feelings—hidden within time obsessions—clock-watching or crunching sleep numbers intractably infects sleep quality, adding to your sleep misery.

Rarely would you find *Sound Sleep*.

Watch Out

Among those with severe mental health symptoms and sleep problems, time monitoring is not only fueled by anxieties and fears, but in turn, time monitoring intensifies these emotions. Time monitoring turns into a figurative deathwatch among those unable to work through their deepest, disabling emotions. They have reached a demoralizing nadir in life in which too much of their time is spent counting down the grains of sand in an hourglass. Such individuals are at high risk for suicidal behavior, because their time obsessions cover up extremely intense, unpleasant emotions. Some are in desperate need of mental health counseling and medication, while others would be wise to seek spiritual counseling.

Breaking the time barrier for these individuals, without professional help, may be ill-advised!

If you have been traumatized once, you are likely to have developed built-in detectors rigorously programmed to alert you to the possibility of it happening again. If it happens again, and you are not ready, this time might be the last time.

Time has infinitely more meaning to someone who has been traumatized; and these individuals can reverse their insomnia much faster when they recognize the deeper meaning of time-monitoring behavior and the emotions associated with it. Instead of wasting energy on their pessimistic, sleep-time relationships, they plug the leak and separate themselves from the menace of time and the damage it does to their sleep quality.

To repeat, psychodynamics may require a mental health professional or pastoral counseling. If you are unwilling to give up the clock, be cautious about proceeding with the next treatment step and consider whether you need professional help breaking the time barrier.

Little Big Step 4

What does time mean to you? Do you really believe you can know how much time is left or that you can control every second of your destiny? No matter how much comfort and security you believe you gain by checking the little clock or the Big Clock, you will never be able to control your sleep with this particular behavior; worse, it can destroy your slumber hour by hour, minute by minute, second by second.

At tonight's *Day Is Done* session, let's add psychodynamic steps to end this self-defeating behavior once and for all. You may wish to learn these steps with the aid of your therapist, and recall your SOLO technique as you start:

- Try your best to link your time monitoring to a particular emotion, even if the only feeling is feeling more "comfortable" looking at the clock:

    Comfort or a sense of control are the most common feelings reported by clock-watchers, and these feelings represent the benefit gained by monitoring time instead of focusing on deeper feelings.

- Next, try to move beyond "comfortable" by guessing what uncomfortable feeling would crop up if the clock were gone:

    Frustration, anxiety, or fear are the most common guesses, and usually one of these three feelings is right on target.

- If you are not skilled in feeling your feelings or emotions, you can still think about them to select the one with the strongest link to your monitoring behavior:

    If you are not sure, do yourself a favor and make a prediction about the single feeling likely to be pushing you to obsess about time.

- Then, on a piece of paper or in the margin, write the name of this feeling:

    If you sense several important feelings or emotions, write the names of these feelings and rank them 1, 2, 3.

- Now, for just a few seconds, try to stop thinking about this process and ask yourself in your heart of hearts if this feeling is the right one:

    Try to sense unequivocally and honestly whether this emotion is part of the process pushing you to watch the clock or crunch sleep numbers.

- At this point in treatment, please notice that these steps do not require you to make any special effort to feel this feeling:

    The goal is to experience a quiet reflection for a minute or less to clarify your sense of certainty about the feeling and your desire to monitor time.

- Your objective is not to spend much time at all feeling these feelings, especially if you believe they might overwhelm you.

    Last, if relevant to your circumstances, now would be the time to consider prayer as another helpful aid in finding closure on the day.

When you complete these steps tonight or for the next few nights, pat yourself on the back. Although you might not initially recognize why these actions count as a big success, your efforts represent the initial psychodynamic steps needed to break the time barrier. It does not matter that you might not know how to work through these feelings yet. Indeed, our focus is to not rush you into spending too much time feeling feelings, because proceeding cautiously is safer for those troubled sleepers whose TFI imbalances minimize feelings and emotions.

Future steps will teach you more advanced techniques on how to work with feelings and emotions. At this point, if you are frustrated in your efforts, take a step back and remember that while time is your enemy, timing is everything.

Sands of Time

Looking at a clock or ruminating about time is a reliable way to ignore feelings. But the longer you ignore them, time obsessions invariably prevent closure so that night after night:

- Your *Day Is Never Done.*
- Your *Wave of Sleepiness* is nonexistent.
- Your mind and body really have no desire to sleep.

Psychodynamic perspectives are powerful and therapeutic: *Knowing exactly what you are dealing with makes it much more possible to deal with it . . . even if it scares you at first.*

The sands of time fall through the hourglass. Are you still gaining something by watching each grain of sand drop through the funnel? If you realize how easily a clock feeds anxieties and worries, you will know that the clock does not provide the comfort or control you seek. Sooner or later, you must accept that you cannot hold back the sands of time by staring down the clock.

If time waits for no one, why should you wait for time?

SLEEP ON IT
An Eye for Your Feelings

QUESTION: The primary purpose of human emotion is to protect you to ensure your survival, safety, and security. The single most important feeling—love—protects you, because without feeling loved or loving someone, you cannot experience real security, you often find yourself in unsafe circumstances, and you may not survive. All emotions serve to protect, but it takes time and reckoning to understand how this process unfolds.

Crossing the street is a clear example in which fear makes you look both ways. If your *TFI System* is out of balance, you may believe that intellect makes you watch passing cars; thinking certainly is part of the reflex keeping you from getting run over. But, if your amygdala (the brain's fear sensor) were damaged, thus erasing your "fear factor," you would lose the motive to look both ways when crossing the street. Head injury patients with damaged amygdalas demonstrate poor judgment when confronted with simulated, dangerous scenarios. They have lost much of their "emotional intelligence."

Feelings provide *Emotional Intel* that leads to greater balance in your *TFI System*. *Emotional Intel* in the example was "passing cars threaten me." Looking both ways means you received and used the *Intel*, an action termed "emotional processing."

Most with *TFI System* imbalances assume they access this information by "thinking about their feelings," but in reality a "feeling" pathway provides more Intel. When you only think about your emotions, you develop lots of theories and speculations about what you're feeling, usually to fit preconceived notions of what you want your feelings to be and what you want the feelings to mean. Sometimes this technique produces useful results if you suffer regularly from too much emotion.

If you think too much—the more common imbalance—you must learn to evaluate feelings from their side of the equation, which produces clearer emotions. These pure feelings course through your body for a few seconds or a few minutes. They come and go. This process sparks surprisingly accurate and highly pragmatic *Emotional Intel* to act upon.

Your heart truly speaks to your mind!

In the heat of the night, *Emotional Intel* proves invaluable in resolving insomnia. Unquestionably, successfully working through troublesome feelings (emotional processing) is more powerful than any sleeping pill ever invented. Despite the purposeful roles that feelings and emotions play, many poor sleepers are confused or nervous about processing feelings because emotion is viewed as a cause of sleeplessness, not the cure for it. Developing one's Emotional Intelligence may prove difficult. If you never tasted key lime pie, no description suffices. To "taste" your emotions, the recipe must suit your taste buds. At this point I must caution you that spending too much time with feelings also might cause a problem. Just like thinking too much, feeling too much creates an imbalance, which may worsen your sleep quality.

So let's pause in our discussion of emotion and recognize that to find the right balance in the *TFI System* of thoughts, feelings, and images, we must examine the component you literally never want to lose sight of.

Imagery is overlooked by troubled sleepers and is rarely broached by health-care providers. Imagery helps change self-defeating learned behaviors, and if your feelings feel stuck, imagery is an ideal way to get them unstuck. Once you train yourself to invoke imagery in your mind's eye, you discover that images serve as a reliable bridge between thoughts and feelings. Having examined your thoughts and feelings, what have you noticed about the pictures in your mind's eye?

COMMENT: The pictures in your mind play a near-miraculous role in solving sleep problems. As a child, you enjoyed picturing things in your mind, including dreams and daydreams. If your family was not enthusiastic about pictures or stories, you may have lost interest in your mind's eye. Or your interests could have waned if your family overemphasized verbal thinking or talking in place of artistic or imaginary things.

We all retain the capacity to picture things. Visualizing behavior is easily engaged when asked for street directions. A picture or a map pops into your mind's eye, supplying roads and landmarks to show the way. The capacity to generate pictures or images is an incredibly powerful tool that can solve problems, make decisions, enhance memory, sort out troublesome feelings, clarify confusing thoughts, rest your brain, and help you fall asleep faster than sleeping pills.

SNOOZE FLASH
Imagery in the Nick of Bed*time*

If your imagery system functions well, and disturbing images rarely pop up, begin using pleasant imagery now at bedtime or in the middle of the night to help you fall or return to sleep.

——— PEARL ———
Make Your Imagery More Powerful
Than the Sandman

Before you use the following instructions, perform the SOLO technique to prime your mind's eye. Pay attention to how fleeting images are as they fly across your mental landscape. Watch them come and go. Many images seem neutral or meaningless; others are pleasant or unpleasant. The most valuable thing to notice is whether you notice images in your mind's eye. If you do not pay attention to the pictures, figure out why. Trauma survivors do not wish to recall the memories of awful experiences, but even those who suffer horrific memories or nightmares can learn to control these images as they balance the *TFI System*.

Find a comfortable place to spend ten to twenty minutes, without interruptions. Place your body in a symmetrical position, sitting or lying, and support your head and neck so they won't slump or roll to one side.

Close your eyes for one minute; notice whether images spontaneously emerge. If they don't, open your eyes, look at something that catches your eye, and stare at it for one minute. Close your eyes again and bring that image into your mind's eye. If it's still difficult, open and close your eyes repetitively until the image emerges, or simply keep your eyes closed for ten straight minutes to see whether any images emerge.

Don't confuse this exercise with trying to develop photographic images in your mind's eye. Perfect imagery is difficult to achieve, and it's not needed to make use of your imagery system or to help you sleep.

Once you notice images, keep your eyes closed for five to ten minutes to expand this exercise in creative ways. Have fun and relive a great vacation, an exhilarating hike in the woods, a satisfying round of golf, your kid's soccer game, going dancing, and so on.

You only need to spend a few minutes each day practicing pleasant imagery, unless you first need more time activating your imagery system. Notice how frequently various images, not to mention thoughts and feelings, come and go during imagery exercises.

PART THREE

PICTURE PERFECT SLEEP
Mind's-Eye Imagery Conquers Insomnia

Leaving Time Behind

You have always possessed a *TFI System*, and coordinating a fully balanced *TFI System* brings enormous gains, regardless of any other treatment steps you attempt. For most troubled sleepers, balance does not come easily. Instead, thinking seems most natural and tilts things away from feelings and images. So we must spend more time learning about images and feelings, the aim of the next two parts of this book.

Now is the time to gain greater precision in working with these other two building blocks of the *TFI System*. Learning to use the whole system is akin to knowing the alphabet of a language. When you group letters together, you make sense of words. When you group thoughts, feelings, and images together, you create a more detailed picture of the specific things that influence your sleep.

Last, and never least, by continuously applying these elements, you soon arrive at a place where you really do want to be asleep, at which time the *Wave of Sleepiness* carries you safely to the shores of *Sound Sleep* and keeps you there as long as needed.

11

Finding Comfort in the Eye of the Storm

New Treatment Targets

Your primary goal is to sleep well all through the night.

To achieve this goal, you would expect no difficulties with falling asleep, staying asleep through the night, or waking up refreshed and rested. While eliminating time-monitoring behavior slows down your brain waves and leads to modest to large improvements in these areas, most poor sleepers also want to learn additional tools to fall asleep rapidly, to stop waking up, and to return to sleep quickly if awakened.

Please make a short list of the factors that prevent you from sleeping through the night. Here's a sample list:

- My mind won't turn off: the wheels are spinning and my thoughts race along.
- I feel tense, keyed up. I feel tired, but I don't feel like I could fall or return to sleep.
- I worry or think about something that happened yesterday, that's happening now, that will happen tomorrow.
- I am anxious or depressed about . . . something.
- I am frustrated, angry, or sad about . . . something.
- My body just cannot get comfortable.
- Mr. Crabapple's dogs are barking.
- The bedroom is too hot [or too cold].

- The bedroom is too dark [or too bright].
- I honestly don't know why I wake up or can't return to sleep.

Maybe you listed other items, but generally these are the most common explanations. These causes are all potential targets, but they are almost always secondary to the overriding problem:

You really do not want to go to sleep or back to sleep because your *Day Is Not Done* . . . which means the *Wave of Sleepiness* is far from shore.

To Sleep or Not to Sleep

Some poor sleepers remain perplexed about the unwitting desire to not be asleep—the desire that serves as the chief engineer of this out-of-control train ride down the tracks of sleeplessness—because most cannot figure out why they wake up at night in the first place. As odd as it sounds, waking up in the middle of the night is a reflection of the same problem—you may not want to be asleep. Just before you awaken, your mind-body decides to remain asleep or to awaken. For various reasons, you "choose" to awaken because at that moment you do not want to be asleep. In nearly all such circumstances, your brain is moving too fast to sleep.

According to this theory:

- If you are anxious in the middle of the night, you may develop this emotion to prevent yourself from sleeping.
- If your thoughts are racing, you are using racing thoughts to prevent yourself from going to sleep or returning to sleep.
- If your body is uncomfortable or antsy (not in significant pain), discomfort "helps" you stay awake—your unsuspected goal.
- You might use the clock, unwittingly, to monitor time and sleep hours to activate your mind and keep yourself awake.

Surely we all agree that anxiety, worries, ruminations, racing thoughts, time obsessions, and discomfort cause you to stay awake. But it is distinctly possible that you generate each of these conditions for the unequivocal objective of preventing your return to sleep, not the other way around. As strange as it sounds, the faster you consider or observe this behavior in yourself (if true), the faster you overcome insomnia.

Even if you are not persuaded by this theory yet, please consider what you would do if it proved to be true. If you really don't want to be asleep when you awaken in the middle of the night, can you imagine the best steps or strategies to get back to sleep? Please give this question a SOLO moment before reading the next little big step.

Little Big Step 5: Invitation to a Slumber Party

If you really do not want to be asleep in the middle of the night, then the fastest possible way to get back to sleep would be to first:

Have a Good Time!

If your day is not done, and you are awake in the middle of the night, then stopping all efforts to sleep is the strongest pill in your medicine chest. The key is to take advantage of your time awake in a way sure to please and satisfy. How you choose to do so proves critical.

"Do I have a good time . . ."

- in bed or somewhere else?
- for a short or a long time?
- that's recreational or productive?

Ideally, it's somewhere besides the bedroom, for a relatively short time frame, and with something recreational or relaxing. In some situations, it's to your advantage to spend a longer time accomplishing a task. The clearest way to try out this strategy is to sit up in bed, immediately give yourself a one-minute SOLO technique, and then honestly say to yourself as appropriate:

"I know right now I am not going to sleep or I am not going back to sleep, because I may not really want to sleep." Then, get out of bed and if possible leave the bedroom, and don't come back until you are ready, willing, and able to sleep.

Tough instructions, right?

Tough, yet extremely powerful and surprisingly comforting.

During your time awake, you must learn to spend absolutely no time thinking about your sleep in any way whatsoever, which also means no time spent checking the time or figuring out how much sleep time is slipping away. Don't even think about solving the riddle of why you woke or why you cannot return to sleep. If your bed and bedroom feel like a torture chamber, then realize here and now how valuable it can be for you to get up out of bed and do something to make you happy, or ideally make you laugh, but at a minimum, bring you comfort, pleasure, or satisfaction:

- Read a book.
- Watch a funny movie.
- Play a computer game.
- Write a letter.
- Play a musical instrument.
- Play solitaire or Sudoku.
- Surf the Net.
- Listen to some enjoyable and relaxing music.
- Above all, forget about sleep and stop trying to sleep.

Under certain conditions, you can clean your house or engage in work. The objective is to enjoy or satisfy yourself. Some people love to clean when no one distracts them; the same holds for certain work-oriented projects, which may be more satisfying alone. It does not matter what you select as long as you picture a reasonable stopping point, usually thirty minutes to two hours. There's no magic to the number of minutes. Most problematic sleepers who successfully overcome middle-of-the-night awakenings report it takes only thirty minutes to two hours to bring back a *Wave of Sleepiness*. Then falling asleep back in your bed is relatively easy, which means don't fall asleep on the sofa or anyplace else. Wait until you return to bed.

Make special use of your time. Instead of believing you are punishing yourself by getting out of bed, appreciate this time and treat yourself well. The *Wave of Sleepiness* is closer to the shore than you imagine. Clear the fog and you'll see it and feel the *Wave*, swirling at your feet.

SLEEP ON IT
Out of Bed, but Not out of Sleep

QUESTIONS: Can you predict how your *TFI System* responds to "get up out of bed and have a good time"? Do you see how the system could help or hurt you in trying out this step?

COMMENT: Most poor sleepers groan, raise their eyebrows, or seem confused about leaving the bed in the middle of the night. "Why should I get out of bed if I'm trying to sleep?" The frozen-to-the-mattress routine is classic sleep quantity thinking, based on "more is more"—more time in bed offers more sleep. Let's divide this reaction into its three TFI parts:

1. *thinking* the idea is irrational, because you need more time in bed to get more sleep;

2. *feeling* confused, irritated, or angry about the very notion of getting out of bed;

3. *picturing* in your mind's eye an awful episode of getting out of bed at night.

Notice how each brain activity could trigger a new cycle of TFIs, steering you away from these instructions or helping you perceive their value.

The *TFI System* is not simplistic, but the following example shows how simply a behavior might be adjusted. Suppose you were trying to finish a novel but found no time to read it. Using the *TFI System*, you might picture yourself reading in the middle of the night, sparking a pleasant feeling about finishing the book. This new feeling of pleasure can replace the frustrated feelings about not sleeping. And these changed images and feelings could influence your thinking: "I just turned something negative into something positive."

You unlearned a "losing sleep over losing sleep" behavior because you chose to "have a good time" reading instead of wasting energy lying in bed, worrying about not sleeping. But there's more: you reemphasize sleep quality, minimize pressure from closure problems, and unlearn the behavior of lying in bed awake, all of which can lead to slower brain waves. Changing thoughts, feelings, and images was the key, a powerful one at that.

─── PEARL ───

A Change in Scenery Might Be All You Need

The complexity of the *TFI System* arises when you doubt that reading in the middle of the night is a fun and healthy alternative to lying in bed awake. Maybe you cannot generate a pleasant picture to see yourself reading peacefully. Or frustrated and angry emotions about losing sleep feel stuck, so you cannot feel positive about getting up from bed.

You could convince yourself that getting out of bed is stupid, outrageous, and torturous, meriting no consideration. You might react strongly to the fool offering this dire instruction. Many physicians and therapists, untrained in delivering this technique, "lose" patients when ample rationale is not offered to bolster confidence. I earnestly want you to know this powerful approach to healthy control over nighttime awakenings. Most troubled sleepers improve with its use within a week or less. The pressing issue is whether your *TFI System* helps or prevents you from considering this option. An imbalanced *TFI System* may close your eyes to it.

In your effort toward balance, don't assume that each TFI element is engaged 33 percent of the time. The system is not about percentages; it's about the healthy flow of TFIs that come and go. If you are lucky enough to know normal sleepers, ask one to describe what goes on in his or her mind and *TFI System* when falling asleep. This information yields a clue to the meaning of balance, especially related to falling asleep. Ask a normal sleeper . . . if you can find one. You'll be super lucky if you find one who describes what happens with the pictures in the mind's eye just at sleep onset.

SNOOZE FLASH

Balancing Acts Bring Fast Relief

If your *TFI System* is stuck, disregard the "get up out of bed" tool for now. By attempting to balance your *TFI System* first, you might return to sleep quite naturally.

12

Puzzling through It All

New Balancing Acts

You are the master of the bed and the bedroom.

If you suffer silently, wide awake, and frozen to your mattress, then you are treating yourself like a prisoner or a slave to bed and bedroom. Your temple of sleep should provide you with the foundation for peace and tranquillity. If every minute you lie awake in bed and fight to sleep, you are letting your power and energy slip out of your hands as surely as if you were tipping a glass of water, pouring out its contents. As problematic as it might be to alter this behavior, you need to give yourself a break from your bed or bedroom to sever the connection between your sleep space and your broken sleep. Breaking this connection slows down your brain waves to get you sleepy again in the middle of the night or when you first try to sleep.

For every thirty minutes awake in bed anxious and frustrated, in only fifteen minutes outside the bedroom you usually gain a small increase in your natural sleepiness. For every minute spent comforting yourself, away from the bedroom, you usually avert about two minutes of emotional pain frozen to your mattress. These minutes add up, and you often discover that a bad night spent in the grips of your torture chamber for two hours could have been consolidated and reversed in a delightful one-hour session reading a collection of funny short stories. After one hour of amusement, your mind-body is prepared to sleep again. You accomplished your objective of getting to sleep in half the time it usually takes and with far less pain than you would ordinarily suffer by sticking to the mattress.

But you must seize the opportunity to enjoy yourself regardless of the inappropriateness of the hour. Through this waking behavior, whatever you choose, you often satisfy an unrecognized need or work through emotions needing attention. Your satisfaction brings comfortable and relaxing feelings, leading to the pleasure of sleepiness. The *Wave* ultimately returns sleep to your blessed bed, which you shall transform into a sacred place of slumber.

Little Big Step 6: Make Plans, Not War

Figuring out what to do in the middle of the night poses some obstacles. You might prefer to give no thought to this problem, because it is so annoying to consider climbing out of bed or leaving the bedroom in the dead of night. If you wait until the witching hour, you could generate more frustrations and never attempt the instructions.

Let's not wait, let's plan. Let's prepare for the middle of the night, maybe tonight, long before such awakenings occur. Foremost, let's figure out behaviors best suited for you. Never discount your creative resources. Start with the SOLO technique as you consider these options:

- Something truly fun, producing laughter, such as an *I Love Lucy* rerun.
- Something truly satisfying, engaging your emotions without over-stimulating you. Novels, short stories, and fiction are great, but not suspense thrillers or mysteries.
- Something truly productive, if time-limited, requiring movement of your body. Cleaning and organizing around the house are great. Writing is remarkably effective, because you are moving your hands with pen or pencil on paper or with a keyboard. You must obtain a sense of accomplishment in thirty minutes to two hours.

It may be valuable to combine any or all these actions (fun, satisfaction, and sense of accomplishment), but the more immediate goal is to pick at least one thing and test it out the next time you wake up at night and cannot return to sleep in less than fifteen minutes. Buy a video, select a book, pull out a deck of cards, or look over your CD collection.

Your goal is to return to the sense of *Day Is Done*, so your mind-body slows down. To produce this feeling, some must work on a project yielding a sense of accomplishment, which then brings closure that may have been missing at bedtime. These individuals run a risk of overstimulation if they select tasks that normally take weeks or months. Think small at 3:00 A.M.

Many professional writers as well as many others who write for work or pleasure find writing for an hour in the middle of the night very satisfying and productive. This work leads to sufficient closure to permit sleepiness back into their minds and bodies.

Puzzle Power

The single best plan for middle-of-the-night awakenings involves laying out a thousand-piece jigsaw puzzle on a card table, to use as needed. The power of the puzzle is worth its weight in golden slumbers, because it directly attacks an imagery imbalance in your *TFI System*, and it balances the entire system to welcome the *Wave of Sleepiness* back into the mind-body. Puzzling as this technique seems, unlocking its mysteries might solve your insomnia in the blink of an eye.

When a person wakes in the middle of the night and cannot return to sleep, the most common concern is stopping mental chatter. A large, thousand-piece jigsaw puzzle not only diagnoses this problem if you are still not aware of your own self-talk, but also it resolves this problem sufficiently to permit you to return to sleep.

How and why are jigsaw puzzles so powerful?

When you start a jigsaw puzzle under insomnia circumstances, you are usually engaged in a fast-brain, verbal-thinking mode. Yet self-talk is not the kind of thinking that solves jigsaw puzzles. You cannot talk yourself into putting pieces together. Instead, you need to expand your mental landscape with imagery.

If you try to think about the pieces instead of seeing the pieces, you become frustrated, often tired, and in rare cases, it induces a brief useless feeling of sleepiness, although it more commonly induces a headache. These changes occur quickly because your brain faces an impossible task. The puzzle piece is begging for visual attention, but your mind is only thinking in words at that moment; the conflict cannot be resolved until you choose to see the pieces.

Consider your experience at a foreign film in which subtitles flash across the screen so fast you must work too hard to keep pace with both the dialogue and the action in the flick. The result is less satisfying because you use too much verbal thinking to understand what's going on.

If you feel frustration or mental fatigue when attempting the thousand-piece jigsaw puzzle, you just diagnosed a lack of balance, in which you think too much and image too little. Don't despair; you can change your ways.

Small Changes

You can change immediately by not looking to solve any particular pair of puzzle pieces. You need to change your perspective and look over the whole picture on top of the puzzle box, which permits you to ease into an imagery mind-set. Then look over puzzle pieces for clues—not solutions—that permit you to group pieces together. Here are ways to form groups:

- edge pieces that "frame" the picture;
- pieces of the same solid color (for example, nearly all dark green);
- pieces with similar patterns of color (for example, dark on one half, lighter on the other);
- pieces with similar themes (for example, white lines of a fence or speckles of leaves from a tree);
- Within each of these groups, find subgroups based on similar or contrasting shapes between or among pieces.

Your task at this point is not about solving or organizing the puzzle, so you should feel a noticeable decrease in pressure. You are learning to use your eyes to look back and forth between the "big picture" and various shapes and shades that match quadrants or sections of the puzzle to ease into a rhythm of using your eyes instead of thinking too much.

As your eyes see the pieces, a truly satisfying and pleasurable experience takes hold of your mind. Instead of thinking about pieces or needing to solve the puzzle, your imagery system perks up, and you experience a new form of "thinking," deemed your visual intelligence system, which slows down your brain activity.

Anything but Puzzling

Once you cluster the pieces, you can try to interlock them. However, when your mind is engaged with imagery, you will see that solutions take a backseat to the visual pleasure. As solutions to the puzzle emerge, you see that they do not emerge from a place of self-talk or work. Images seen through your eyes link pieces together without your talking about these connections in your head. You can have thoughts about certain pieces, but most of your mental capacity figures out the pictures within the picture in a pleasurable and satisfying way.

When you overcome your early frustrations by activating imagery, you quickly recognize that you are using your mind in a new way—which as you are about to learn is similar to the way your mind falls asleep.

Soon the puzzle experience becomes anything but puzzling. It's fun, satisfying, and once into it, you feel a sense of accomplishment, sometimes by putting just two pieces together. The jigsaw puzzle strategy may motivate you to use jigsaw puzzles before bedtime to activate imagery or by day to relax or to remind you of the invaluable "slowing" impact of imagery.

Puzzling Through

If you find the experience frustrating after ten minutes, in most cases you are still engaging in too much self-talk. Persistent self-talk means this habit is deeply ingrained, but it also may reflect anxiety or fear about letting your mind delve into feelings and images. In the worst case, self-talk might be replaced by a blank mind with no thoughts or pictures. A blank mind usually signals concerns about what might emerge from your imagery system. You may be concerned that images will provoke unpleasant feelings. A therapist could prove invaluable here.

Here's another step to try first. Hold a single puzzle piece in front of your face. Stare at it as if memorizing its content, then close your eyes and see the piece in your mind's eye. Repeat this step several times; open and close your eyes until you see the pattern of the piece. It is not necessary to see color. Once you see some of the piece in your mind's eye, repeat this step with another piece for about ten more pieces. If this procedure still doesn't work, try it with a few photos of loved ones, the viewing of which should break through the self-talk, if nothing else will. Once you see pictures of loved ones in your mind's eye, move back to the individual puzzle pieces and then to the puzzle.

The key is to use your eyes in every way imaginable to bring your mind into a new state of consciousness. You may want to compare pieces for shades of color, nuances of shape, or similarities of pattern. Using your eyes to explore puzzle distinctions turns off the self-talk button and turns on the balance in your *TFI System*. Balance arises because imagery has a specific capability of diffusing excessive thoughts and feelings.

The jigsaw puzzle approach is an advanced technique that leads to satisfying breakthroughs, because imagery appears to directly and rapidly engage the right side of the brain. In extremely severe insomniacs or severe psychiatric patients, we often encounter extreme left-brain, overly analytic coping styles that dismiss or reject cognitive behavioral therapy (CBT) and psychodynamic solutions. Instead, these same individuals may make great strides using the puzzle technique.

As a bonus to these severe cases as well as others, imagery-induced balance often helps you feel your *Day Is Done*, which then generates the *Wave of Sleepiness* to carry you in no time at all to the land of Nod.

SLEEP ON IT
Imagine That!

QUESTION: Few normal sleepers pay attention to sleep; they just let it happen. When questioned, though, normal sleepers almost universally report falling asleep in a surprisingly routine way, best explained through the *TFI System*.

First, the sleeper notices a feeling of sleepiness at a point in the evening, signaling bedtime, or some fight off this feeling, letting it emerge when the head hits the pillow. Next, in bed, thoughts or feelings emerge, usually of low intensity. Thoughts could be about anything and might start out at a greater clip than seems conducive to sleep. Soon thoughts drift into a realm very different from waking patterns, turning weird, as in "the ice cream truck's plumbing cannot harvest the garden," which you might not recall, but some normal sleepers spot this irrational thinking and recognize sleep in the offing.

Feelings at bedtime are mostly about comfort. The bed feels supportive and relaxing; the sheets feel pleasantly cool or warm. The repositioning of the pillow feels comfortable for head or neck. The body gives up its need for action; rest is welcomed into arms and legs and torso and head. Sleepy feelings predominate, compared to feelings of tiredness or fatigue, and ultimately you feel a beautiful *Wave* washing over your mind.

Last, and never least, the pictures in your mind serve as the gateway through which you embark on your stay over in Nod. As the normal sleeper notices thoughts drifting and feelings comforting, imagery emerges on center stage. The pictures, often as "dreamlets," appear in the mind's eye, yielding "visual pleasure" akin to getting lost in a work of art, although weird or irrational content emerges, too. Some describe it as rapidly changing "moving pictures." As images increase, thoughts and feelings recede into the background, your brain activity slows down, and then you fall asleep. If you "watch" yourself fall asleep, images are the last thing you recall.

When you carefully review this progression, you notice that falling asleep is about letting TFIs "come and go." You might be surprised to discover that you can easily repeat these steps yourself. However, you may not know how to repeat these steps night after night.

Why the lack of consistency?

COMMENT: The most obvious barrier to this natural bedtime progression is an imbalanced *TFI System*, developed through learned behaviors of thinking too much or, in fewer cases, of feeling too much. When sleep beckons, you cannot bring your motor to a low and smooth idle, and no imagery emerges. For those who find it relatively easy to activate imagery at bedtime, you can treat your sleeplessness tonight. Just close your eyes and let the picture show emerge.

More complex reasons underlie imbalances in the *TFI System* for troubled sleepers with mental health concerns, who think too much to purposely avoid unpleasant feelings or images. Among trauma survivors, too much thinking holds back a flood of unpleasant images such as nightmares. Although these examples reflect learned behaviors, the triggering mechanism is more intense due to a past traumatic event. These intense, unpleasant feelings or images all but guarantee a lack of balance.

The *Wave of Sleepiness* is nowhere to be found for these highly troubled sleepers who are left instead with the *tides of sleeplessness*. In the worst scenario, you anticipate the problem of unpleasant feelings or images, so upon lying down, the volume of self-talk increases acutely, preventing feelings or images from creeping up unexpectedly. This type of blockage is severe and requires greater effort and commitment to learn imagery techniques, and it usually requires simultaneous work on your emotions.

———— PEARL ————
Your Imagination Solves Almost Any Sleep Puzzle

Now that you understand the power of imagery and its key role in getting you to sleep, you must determine whether you can activate this essential *TFI System* component. You can use imagery for falling asleep and for waking use as well.

If you have not used pleasant imagery at bedtime, please add this to your routine, unless you struggle with unpleasant images such as nightmares. Whether or not you suffer from unpleasant images, everyone should attempt the next step. You may need to go slowly, but in our experience, even severely traumatized individuals can complete this task.

Begin with a SOLO technique, then select something in your home you wish to change, preferably something simple, not in desperate need of change. The best example is furniture you would be curious to rearrange, but there is no pressing need to do so. Planning a remodel is too intense and stressful for this step. You could also choose things such as combing your hair a new way, moving your pet's food or water bowl, making your bed differently in the morning, or reorganizing your desk. Pick something neutral that does not trigger strong emotions.

Spend five to ten minutes with eyes closed; see if you can picture changes for this theoretical task. Do not attempt the imagery with the belief that you must change something. This step only needs to teach you how to appreciate the dynamic nature of imagery. Pay special attention to how thoughts, feelings, and images come and go during your imagery exercise. This flow is normal, and cultivating the ability to let TFIs come and go brings your system into balance.

If you find the exercise easy, try it out on several ideas for change in your home or work.

13

Imaginary Sleep Friends

Imagine Sleep

The human imagery system is one of the most advanced components of the human mind.

Few problematic sleepers recognize the power of imagery. Tapping your imagery system helps overcome sleep problems faster than the time it takes to request a prescription from your doctor, maybe faster than the drive to your pharmacy. You can activate an imagery system in less than five minutes of practice on the first attempt. You can also respond to middle-of-the-night awakenings by picturing pleasant imagery instead of getting up.

Imagery is so powerful because it slows down brain waves and recruits the *Wave of Sleepiness*. One caveat: until you reenergize this natural capacity, leaving the bed when not sleepy is still prudent.

Eyes Front

When first attempting imagery, many troubled sleepers believe that pictures should emerge without thoughts or feelings intervening. Yet, imagery work for sleep problems has nothing to do with seeing things as photographs in your mind's eye. Imagery, just like thoughts or feelings, is a dynamic process, changing with situations, coming and going.

Please conjure up your capacity to provide directions to a favorite restaurant. Traveling the route in your mind to spot landmarks along the way works well, and as you relate this information to the listener, you must use words (the verbal way to express thought). In the process, don't be surprised when a feeling crops up, "I remember eating a tasty Caesar salad there, which makes me hungry for one right now."

Our aim is not to generate a state of pure imagery, which is nearly impossible to achieve. From practical experience, you know that your waking visual system often relishes sunsets with some intervening mental chatter. Balance does not mean excluding an element; it means balancing TFIs.

Some believe their imagery systems are completely out of their control, but that belief often arises from not having paid much attention to imagery in everyday life. With the following exercises you can learn to manipulate imagery day and night, which dramatically increases your chances of balancing your *TFI System*. If you are struggling with imagery, these exercises prove critical to gaining confidence and momentum. Some need to work with their eyes open before practicing in the mind's eye.

Little Big Step 7: The Eyes Have It

Many imagery paths are possible. Use your eyes to see in front of you, or let awareness move you from the "self-talk" to the "mind's eye" mode:

- *Coloring book*: Color pictures with meaning, value, or appeal. Perhaps your drawings can serve as presents for your kids or other children.
- *Crossword puzzle*: Surprisingly, this technique works if clues trigger images in your mind's eye. If it triggers more self-talk, avoid this approach.
- *Tape and view a PBS nature special*: Notice how these shows compare to most TV. Showing nature's beauty with scant narration yields appealing and relaxing imagery.
- *Rubik's Cube*: If you think about the colored squares, it won't help. Whether or not you solve the cube, the key is to engage your mind with colors and use your visual/imagery system to align squares as best you can.
- *Picture books*: The great, unrecognized value of "coffee table books." Look at the pictures, gather in the details, and let your mind wander over the beauty or intricate images. Visual pleasure is there to devour.

In addition to eyes-on techniques, there are tricks to recruit other senses to fine-tune and enjoy your mind's eye:

- *Guided imagery tapes*: These programs walk through pleasant scenes, such as a garden or a beach. They run ten minutes or longer and help you relax during the day. Use them near or at bedtime to turn on your imagery.
- *Make your own tapes*: Select a pleasant scene, write down a brief script, then read it into a tape player. If a friend or a loved one possesses a soothing voice, let that person read it. Put lots of pauses from five seconds to a minute into the narrative to remove any pressure to "follow" the script.
- *Music CDs*: Many have fond memories of falling asleep listening to music. It works on imagination to quiet down self-talk. Radio music with commercial interruptions is not advised, unless low-key. As you learned to see jigsaw puzzle pieces, learn to hear the music in your mind's ear, which can recruit the *Wave* or activate your imagery.
- *Aroma lamps and aromatherapy*: Your sense of smell relates to emotions and memory. Certain scents, fragrances, or aromas induce feelings of comfort and security or pleasant memories, which activate your imagery.

Here are some unusual tricks to stop self-talk and permit imagery:

- *Eyes open in pitch-black bedroom*: If you sleep in a darkened room with little or no light, sometimes self-talk decreases just by opening your eyes in the darkness. You see next to nothing, and soon your eyes grow too heavy to stay open; it's tiring to look at nothing. Each time you close them, self-talk may return. If you keep holding them open, seeing "nothing," slowly but surely the self-talk ceases, and your eyes become drowsy, then sleepy. Imagery then enters the mind's eye.
- *Repositioning your tongue*: Place your tongue between your teeth while gently bracing but not biting down. This trick is taught to those who learned to read by saying each word inside the mind, which slows down reading. The tongue between your teeth decreases self-talk and yields a bonus of extending the tongue muscles forward. This extension opens the back of the throat, permitting easier breathing, a highly desirable bedtime experience. Lodging the tip of your tongue just above the gum ridges behind the front teeth produces the same effects.

Near bedtime, many other activities can be attempted, such as doodling, drawing, board games, string games, and a host of other children's games. Whenever working with your eyes open, close your eyes from time to time to see if visual images creep in. Once images easily enter the mind's eye, you are very close to sleep. Whether or not you choose to get out of bed or leave the bedroom, you must develop the confidence to turn on your imagery and let your mind's eye wander down the path to sleep.

If you were paying careful attention to this last point, you noticed that sleepiness was not mentioned. Amazingly, some poor sleepers, despite blocking their *Wave*, can engage imagery alone to take them to sleep—without any obvious sleepiness. The ideal scenario occurs when you spend time with imagery, soon find yourself sleepy, and then take both your sleepiness and your imagery to bed. This combination more reliably slows down your brain.

Closure Envy

Normal sleepers have the best of both worlds when it comes to sensing the *Day Is Done* or receiving the *Wave of Sleepiness*. You could call it a hat trick, because the imagery gateway is wide open to them as well. None of these three closure experiences requires conscious effort. Because these normal sleepers slow themselves down at bedtime, presleep experiences chauffeur them straight to sleep. Remarkably, when their routines change after a stressful day, at least one of these elements helps to maintain their uncanny knack of sleeping soundly through the night.

Here's how they do it. If they don't feel sleepiness, they have a clocklike capacity to sense that the day is done, which creates a vacuum into which sleepiness fills the void, even though just seconds or minutes beforehand, sleepiness was nowhere in sight. Amazingly, the reverse experience can unfold as well: the normal sleeper may not feel like the day is done, but at a point in the evening, she suddenly experiences the *Wave* that signals the day must be done, which she easily accepts and goes to bed. Last, if the first two elements are missing in action, many normal sleepers still go to bed, and within seconds or minutes, if their *TFI System* is well balanced, they move quickly through the sequence of random thoughts, comfortable feelings, and imagery on their way to dreamland. These sleepers are truly blessed and may not even know to count their blessings while some of us count sheep.

Problematic sleepers need to appreciate these lessons from normal sleepers' experiences. The troubled sleeper needs to realize that these three processes are intertwined, yet each one can be separately recruited in conscious ways to pull the other two elements along for the ride.

You want to invest a lot of time and energy on imagery, because in the heat of the night if you recruit images into your mind's eye to replace just some of your self-talk or unpleasant feelings, it frequently and instantaneously slows the brain and permits you to go or return to sleep when lying in bed. Arguably, imagery is the tool with the greatest precision and possibly the greatest power to cure insomnia.

Many people wonder about what they are supposed to image at bedtime. The answer is anything, because it usually doesn't matter what you start with. In a short time, you will see your mind's eye naturally wandering through an array of images, most of which you'll never recall when you fall asleep within minutes.

For those with disturbing images during the day or the night, this chapter's Sleep on It section proves especially informative and helpful.

SLEEP ON IT
A Picture Is Worth a Thousand Verbs

QUESTION: Unpleasant images are the largest stumbling blocks to learning imagery. Troubled sleepers, particularly trauma survivors and those with mental health concerns, learn to shut down their imagery systems to suppress disturbing dreams or troubling memories. These imagery problems may require professional help while you work on the next set of exercises. Do you suffer from unpleasant images?

COMMENT: Nearly all people report some unpleasant images. The key to dealing with these pictures (although not necessarily all negative images) is to appreciate and harness the dynamic of your imagery system, which permits the coming and going of TFIs.

The natural state of the mind is for these brain activities to continuously present new ideas and opportunities for the next thing you are going to do, think about, or work on in your waking or dreaming life. Because you have goals and ambitions, you listen to only a few of these elements in the course of the day.

Everyone possesses some capacity to let TFIs come and go because it is not humanly possible to address every thought, feeling, and image experienced during the day. Your imagery system, as a part of this larger *TFI System*, also lets images come and go! Letting images come and go seems difficult to a trauma survivor, but if you had success with the previous change exercise in the last Sleep on It section, then you should have witnessed firsthand that a fair number of images came and went when picturing the rearranged furniture, for example. Once you appreciate this potential, it is rewarding to see unpleasant or other negative images receding without your lifting an imaginary finger.

When you reach this stage in your imagery development, you realize the picture show in your mind's eye is not only free, but scary movies are often just short subjects, brief glimpses of stuff that might quickly recede into the background. When bad images feel more like previews of coming attractions, then more is at stake, and more must be done to prevent them from turning into feature-length presentations.

Nightmares and disturbing dreams are some of the most troubling forms of imagery, and these unwelcome visitors feel utterly uncontrollable. Nightmares are a common cause of poor sleep, because they provoke troubled dreamers to put off their bedtimes to later at night to avoid sleeping and the dreams that eventually follow.

Our research team specializes in treating nightmares in all sufferers, including individuals exposed to sexual assault, other criminal assaults, or disasters; 9/11 survivors; and war veterans, as well as those without any mental health concerns. From our work, we have shown a high likelihood that the overwhelming majority of chronic nightmares become entrenched as unavoidable learned behaviors. In an article our group published in the *Journal of the American Medical Association* in 2001, a randomized controlled study showed that an imagery exercise—imagery rehearsal therapy—reduces disturbing dreams without additional therapy or medication.

———— PEARL ————
Imagery Rehearsal Therapy Treats Bad Dreams and Nightmares

Imagery rehearsal therapy (IRT) can be used to treat bad dreams, to address other unpleasant images that crop up during the daytime, and to overcome disturbing images at bedtime that prevent sleep. IRT is a natural extension of your previous efforts at "changing images."

Here's how it works. Start by recognizing that an unpleasant image has emerged in your mind's eye. As soon as you recognize the presence of the image, use your imagery skill to change the

image to some other picture of your choosing. If you are working on a bad dream, you could do the exercise when you wake
in the middle of the night, or you could do the exercise in the
morning if you recall the nightmare. Change the bad dream into
a "new dream."

Next, spend a few seconds to several minutes rehearsing the
new picture or images you created. If you have trouble with the
old, unpleasant image cropping up, see if you can let that negative image come and go. Then return to your new image and
spend time developing that picture and any story you want to go
along with it. Soon you will appreciate that you possess more
control over the images in your mind's eye than you thought. For
the technique to be effective, you need only work on changing
one or two nightmares each week. Trying to work on too many
bad dreams is unnecessary and may slow progress.

Most nightmare sufferers report decreases in their bad
dreams in about two weeks, and a large majority report solid
and sustained improvements within two months. Once the disturbing dreams decrease, you may only need to practice IRT a
few times per week to reinforce the new habit of not having
nightmares.

Imagery is not an uncontrollable function, although when
first working on imagery exercises, things might feel out of control or overwhelming. Please practice imagery in short bursts initially, such as a few seconds or a few minutes each day. If you
have difficulty moving forward, consider our audio series and
treatment workbook *Turning Nightmares into Dreams*, available
at www.nightmaretreatment.com or www.sleepdynamictherapy
.com, for more in-depth instruction and discussion of IRT.

Once you appreciate the power of imagery, you realize how
imagery can promote balance in the whole *TFI System*, because
imagery is a perfect bridge to travel back and forth between your
thoughts and feelings.

PART FOUR

SLEEP SECRETS OF EMOTIONAL INTEL
Feel Your Way to Better Sleep

Moving Forward and Deeper

Nearing the halfway point, are you halfway home to *Sound Sleep*?

Most troubled sleepers achieve sizable gains by breaking the time barrier, employing the "have a good time" philosophy, when necessary, and consistent use of imagery skills. Yet two deeply entrenched barriers may still prevent you from attaining dramatic gains in sleep quality:

- Specific inhibitors to the feeling of sleepiness, which block the *Wave* from coming ashore;
- TFI imbalances caused by imagery issues or, more often, distressing feelings or emotions.

These five chapters are very intense. You might need a week or longer to work on any one. You will want to reread this section to properly comprehend and apply the instructions on managing your emotions.

A Poor Response May Bring Hopeful News

In my clinical experience, most troubled sleepers suffer physical sleep problems from sleep breathing or movement disorders that go unrecognized for years, because physicians and therapists rarely suspect them or refer patients for sleep testing. In parts six and seven, you'll learn how these conditions are very treatable. For now, never lose sight of this prospect: the absence of large, sustainable improvements in sleep quality—following psychological treatments, especially after using emotion-based therapies—may be a reliable sign of an underlying and untreated physical sleep disorder.

14

Only You Can Prevent Sleepiness

Balance Sheets

The *TFI System* is naturally balanced and takes years to become unbalanced.

This seemingly difficult juggling task appears insurmountable until you consider the analogy of riding a bicycle. When you first ride, it is difficult because you must accomplish three things:

1. think about where you want the bike to go;
2. feel your body supply energy through pedaling;
3. see a point in the distance to keep your equilibrium as you move.

If you do not attend to all three elements, you do not ride long without falling, hitting something, or injuring yourself. It remains difficult until three things occur:

1. pick a spot ahead on which to focus your eyes (visual images);
2. keep pedaling unless it's time to brake (feeling your body);
3. think about your surroundings to bike safely (thinking).

When all three actions take hold, the *TFI System* finds balance, and riding is easy if not instinctual. Never discount your capacity to balance the *TFI System*. It's doable, but for most troubled sleepers certain TFI components lie dormant in daily situations and circumstances. Know now that your

TFI System comes into balance most rapidly by engaging your feelings and emotions.

Catch the Wave

In Sleep Dynamic Therapy (SDT), the most pragmatic way to discuss feelings is to understand three specific ways in which feelings and emotions interfere with the *Wave of Sleepiness*:

1. blocking the *Wave* when you want to sleep;
2. moving the *Wave* to the wrong time of day;
3. reducing the *Wave* to a period too short to help.

As the best example, the presence of intense feelings at bedtime—a lack of emotional closure—represents a clear sign your mind and body do not want to be asleep. Your *Day Is Not Done* and, no surprise, your *Wave of Sleepiness* is lost at sea.

Nightmares and traumatic experiences shed more than a night-light on this mystery, because they promote disturbing feelings that erase feelings of sleepiness. Bad dreams are unwelcome visitors triggering classic learned behaviors in which the eager-to-sleep sleeper enters the bedroom yet grows wide awake, fearful of another attack. Staying awake offers control, so the nightmare sufferer "chooses" not to sleep. Emotions of fear or anxiety block the *Wave*.

In the aftermath of stressful or traumatic events, jittery feelings arise at bedtime—a time of vulnerability—because safety, security, or survival could be at stake. After checking locks, installing an alarm, or purchasing a weapon, the last defense is staying awake instead of sleeping. When you earnestly believe your life or safety is on the line, sleep seems irrational because you relinquish your ability to monitor threats, and ultimately your ability to defend yourself. Whether a trauma survivor recognizes it or not, fear or anxiety blocks the *Wave* from coming ashore.

The Unwavering Wave

Trading sleep for safety, security, or survival is a no-brainer once the threat (nightmares or trauma, for example) grows strong enough, but over time, a troubled sleeper no longer perceives how the *Wave* was corrupted. Indeed, most poor sleepers do not perceive or understand the exact mechanism of this corrupting process.

Do you see how the inability to feel the *Wave* is the exact spot where things go wrong?

Do you realize the amazing fact that the unwavering *Wave of Sleepiness* is almost certainly still there, hiding, as it were, beneath other waves of feelings or emotions? Somewhere inside your mind and body, the *Wave* is eager to emerge, but it cannot wash ashore because you do not want to be asleep.

Many medical experts do not support this view. They believe that a large proportion of troubled sleepers cannot experience sleepiness as normal sleepers do, that somehow their brain waves are genetically programmed to speed up and corrupt the *Wave*. In their view, the answer is to prescribe a pill to induce sleepiness.

Our clinical and research experiences are much different. Greater than 95 percent of our patients report some sleepiness; however, they often experience it at the wrong time of day, in situations not conducive to sleeping, or for intervals too short to let themselves fall or stay asleep. Even among those who declare they don't feel sleepy at all, it seems as if they forgot how to notice this experience, not that they have lost it.

If you learn to spot the factors—most often, very precise feelings or emotions—that prevent the *Wave* from crashing gently on your shore, you can bring sleepiness back to the right place (bedroom), at the right time (bedtime), and for the right amount of time (sleep time).

Little Big Step 8: A Beacon to Light Your Way

Now you must examine how feelings and emotions block the *Wave*. This step shifts us back to daytime, where once and for all we must know the distinctions among three critical feelings:

1. sleepiness;
2. tiredness;
3. fatigue (chronic tiredness).

For the next few days, monitor these three feelings. Know how they feel, when you feel them, and what causes you to feel them. To make rapid progress, notice where you feel them in your mind or body. These next steps are more involved than anything else offered to this point, so start with a strong SOLO effort.

Make six observations a day. Here's a BEACON to light your way for when to do the steps:

1. B = in **B**ed, right after waking up in the morning;
2. E = **E**ating breakfast but before drinking caffeinated beverages;
3. A = shortly before **A**.M. ends (before noon), during a lull;
4. C = usual **C**atnap time, one or two hours after lunch;
5. O = **O**ver the dinner meal;
6. N = early in the **N**ight, one or two hours after dinner.

On each occasion, ask yourself the next eight questions. Once you get the hang of things, it takes less than a minute to run through them all. During the first few trials, please walk or crawl through the questions, which could take five minutes.

- Do I feel sleepy?
  Could I actually fall asleep or doze off if circumstances permitted?
- Do I feel tired?
  Am I feeling low energy but without the desire to sleep?
- Do I feel fatigued?
  Can I distinguish between chronic tiredness (fatigue) and being tired after, say, cleaning the house or mowing the lawn?
- Do I need to take action for any of these feelings?
  If not, what happens to these feelings during the day?

Nearly all poor sleepers attempting these steps will experience some sleepiness. However, if you cannot tap into this precise feeling, chances are you turned sleepiness into feelings of tiredness or fatigue. This mystery is deeply entwined in the special feelings called emotions, which, if left unsolved, push you to believe that pills are the best insomnia therapy.

A Crowd of Feelings

The *Wave of Sleepiness* is a pure feeling of sleepiness. When tiredness or fatigue enters the equation, sleepiness is tainted or crowded out. Pure sleepiness easily puts you to sleep, but sleepiness polluted by other feelings yields little sleep.

Corrupted sleepiness, then, is at the heart of the matter, and the damage to pure sleepiness is best explained by the following equations:

- Sleepiness + anxiety = tiredness or fatigue.
- Sleepiness + frustration = tiredness or fatigue.
- Sleepiness + anger = tiredness or fatigue.
- Sleepiness + stress = tiredness or fatigue.

- Sleepiness + worry = tiredness or fatigue.
- Sleepiness + fear = tiredness or fatigue.
- Sleepiness + anxiety disorder = tiredness or fatigue or worse anxiety disorder.
- Sleepiness + depressive disorder = tiredness or fatigue or worse depressive disorder.
- Sleepiness + PTSD = tiredness or fatigue or worse PTSD.

And in contrast to all the above:

- Sleepiness + nothing else = sleepiness.

SLEEP ON IT
Unsticking Stuck Feelings

QUESTIONS: Throughout this book and in any encounters you may have with sleep specialists, you are constantly bombarded with questions about daytime fatigue and sleepiness. Invariably we ask how these symptoms affect daytime functioning. Now we must turn things around and show you how to work with these daytime feelings of fatigue and sleepiness to understand and solve your sleep problems.

To take advantage of this new perspective, you must realize that every time you feel one of these feelings, it is offering you an enormous amount of information. And the key to unraveling this information is based on your ability to recognize whether you are fighting with feelings of sleepiness, tiredness, or fatigue. Do you fight these feelings? Do you caffeinate them away? Do you battle with them in other ways?

COMMENT: At times it's sensible to fight these feelings because your priorities exceed your low energy state. You must overcome low energy to get the job done. But if you keep fighting on a regular basis, you are less likely to receive the message about what's wrong with your sleep.

The best example is the use of caffeine to fight off low energy. Our aim here is not to discontinue drinking coffee, tea, or sodas, because an enormous number of problematic sleepers drive or work more safely by using caffeine. Our aim is to realize how actively you fight with yourself by fighting off tiredness, fatigue, or sleepiness by self-medicating with caffeine. If you are a caffeine user, chances are high that some sleepiness lurks in your mind-body. But, with regular caffeine use, you have blunted your capacity to experience sleepiness.

If you have been fighting with sleepiness by medicating it away with caffeine, do you see how it would add to your confusion about sleepiness at bedtime? Under safe circumstances, while not driving a car or engaging in other potentially dangerous activities, you can discontinue caffeine to see if your sleepiness emerges.

Once you recognize a sleepy feeling, notice whether you desire a nap. Whether you doze is irrelevant. The key is to recognize that you can experience sleepiness during the day or evening, which means you can learn to move this feeling to bedtime or nighttime.

———— PEARL ————
Find a Home for Your Sleepiness at Bedtime

As you pay closer attention to feelings of sleepiness, relish the experience. Any sort of drowsy feeling is what you aim for in these exercises to show you what you want and need at bedtime. Usually you'll notice that sleepiness feelings are too short-lived or at the wrong time to help solve sleep problems at night. That's okay for now, because at least you reconfirmed your ability to feel sleepiness.

In many situations you notice you literally fight with low energy feelings. Here's a quick SOLO bonus to try if you observe yourself feeling tired and notice you are trying to ward it off. Instead of keeping up the battle, stop fighting, and let the tired feeling course through your body. Often, tired feelings come and go. When you stop fighting and let yourself feel tired in your body, tiredness decreases noticeably and sometimes goes away. This exercise is less useful for fatigue (chronic tiredness), but to reiterate, it also helps discern sleepiness.

Although many poor sleepers make progress by distinguishing among these three feelings, usually your progress is slowed when a missing piece of the puzzle is not recognized. The missing piece is almost always another unrecognized feeling or emotion, like those listed previously, which interfere with efforts to feel the *Wave*.

Everyone agrees that intense emotions conflict with sleep. What is surprising is how few people understand the technical factors that cause emotions to prevent or disrupt sleep. When you feel intense emotions at night, the following are nearly always true:

- Your *Day Is Not Done.*
- You really do not want to sleep.
- Your *Wave of Sleepiness* is corrupted.

These cardinal sleep truths speak to the purpose and nature of human emotions and reveal how and why human emotions rob us of *Sound Sleep.* If you suffer from tainted sleepiness feelings, the solution requires more than overcoming self-talk or using imagery. Now you must turn your attention to the cluster of feelings known as emotions.

15

Emotional Bedbugs
That Bite

Emotional Intelligence

Human emotion is a trustworthy, reliable, and invaluable servant, because human emotions spring from within to serve and protect you.

If you do not pay attention to the warnings, advice, and information embedded in your emotions, they tenaciously repeat themselves until you sign the receipt confirming delivery. Without attending to essential *Emotional Intel*, especially from intense emotions, sleep eludes you unless you use medications. Lingering emotions almost always have a message for you, which, if ignored, prevents closure on the day and corrupts the *Wave of Sleepiness*.

Human emotions represent a compelling, accessible, and nearly inexhaustible early, middle, and late warning system, yet most troubled sleepers, especially those describing difficulties falling asleep or returning to sleep, are confused about this critical component of the *TFI System*. Many insomniacs show their confusion in three ways:

1. a lack of appreciation or understanding of the precise nature of emotions and thus the inability to specifically identify or name emotional experiences;
2. a lack of dexterity or skillfulness in how to feel emotions in the body, often leading to fear or anxiety about having to feel any emotions, even pleasant ones;

3. partial or total ignorance of healthy emotional processing; *Emotional Intel* is routinely ignored, causing feelings to linger well beyond their welcome.

These three problem areas mirror the essential three steps (listed here as one of many possible sequences) required to work through emotions:

1. Identify a feeling (give a specific name to it).
2. Feel the feeling (sense it somewhere in your body).
3. Process the feeling (permit the feeling to come and go).

To use each of these steps successfully, we must first clear up some confusion about emotions, as in the following discussion on anxiety, a topic of great interest and importance to most insomnia patients.

What Is Anxiety?

This set of questions is routinely asked of insomnia patients in our clinics.

First question: "What is anxiety?" Most troubled sleepers do not instinctively reply, "It's a feeling or an emotion." They must be coached, because many call anxiety "worry" or "stress" or indicate that anxiety occurs only in their minds, not their bodies. When reminded that it is a feeling, most still perceive it as mental only.

Second question: "Where do you feel anxiety in your body?" Most patients look perplexed, as if they never heard the question before. To coach them, we add, "and what does anxiety feel like?" Now they pause to "*think* about their feelings," because their answers are not based on paying attention to the body. Some cannot reply, but many mention "tightness in the chest," "lump in the throat," or "queasy stomach," while most insist on racing thoughts, seeing anxiety as just mental.

Third question: "How do you process this feeling . . . how do you work through it to make it go away?" If they are not offered the second part, few grasp the question. Even with the second part, most reply, "I don't know." Another common reply is, "I guess that's what the medication's supposed to do," to which we ask whether it works; the answer is usually, "yes, it works somewhat" and rarely, "yes, it cured my anxieties."

Last Steps First

Most troubled sleepers understand intellectually the first two steps of working with emotions—they can think about naming a feeling and feeling a feeling. But the end result—emotional processing—is the sticking point, because they do not appreciate how emotions come and go. They worry that emotions are coming to spend the night as unwelcome visitors. Or they only understand emotions with phrases, such as "I'm stressed," "I'm anxious," or "I'm depressed," all of which convey more often than not a nagging, chronic sense of unpleasant, ill-defined feelings, which are not the precise emotions you must learn to work with to cleanse your *Sleepiness Wave*.

To overcome this confusion, we must embark on a journey in which you must know your destination long before you head down the path. Although we soon return to the steps for identifying and feeling feelings, let's jump ahead to the last step: emotional processing.

Little Big Step 9: Emotional Processing Inventory

It is crucial to take an inventory of your emotional processing patterns. Most problematic sleepers discover that they deal with emotions by *not* dealing with them. Some think about feelings instead of feeling them as their best way to work with emotions. The following material offers the most common, indirect ways in which adults learn to work with or fight (avoid) working with feelings. Review this material, identify patterns fitting your experience, and recall how you learned these ways. Almost always, you learned them from your parents, siblings, or less often from friends or relatives present in childhood or adolescence. While you might imagine you learned these patterns as adults, usually you can unravel a thread to the past to explain some of your behavior.

These patterns are not exclusively healthy or unhealthy. Many are reasonable things to use, up to a point, but they range from highly effective to highly ineffective ways to process emotions. Some are decidedly dangerous and harmful if used at all. Most people use combinations of these behaviors. You may know other patterns, but those listed are some of the most common among sleep patients.

Never lose sight of the fact that working directly with your feelings is almost always a superior way to process your emotions compared to any of the following indirect techniques:

- **Stuffing your emotions** so your body becomes tense and on guard, as if wearing armor, to fight (defend) against feeling any emotion at all or to use the armor to feel emotions faintly. Among troubled sleepers, this classic form of inadequate emotional processing leads to racing thoughts and ruminations day or night. Individuals of above-average intelligence are susceptible to this pattern, which explains the high prevalence of this style in the high-end academic world, where intense pressure to develop intellectual skills turns students and professors into emotional paupers. As "stuffing" sets in, individuals become so used to being tense, they no longer perceive the *tension* and imagine they are *relaxed*, as they cannot distinguish between the two feelings.

- **Pacifying your emotions** with television, movies, the Internet, or music by engaging these entertainment vehicles not just to be entertained but also to wash away emotions through the programming on the tube, theater, computer, or through lyrics and melodies. Information gathered through media and the Internet may be valuable, but taken to extremes, it reflects an attempt to wash away emotions. Many people using these techniques feel "bored," which is a deceptive feeling, conjured up to avoid dealing with other feelings.

  The TV experience may corrupt or limit natural visual or imagery skills, particularly if you are a passive viewer. Your eyes grow accustomed to fast-paced, rapidly changing sequences, which weakens your capacity to use or focus your eyes in the real world or your mind's eye. You stop seeing things, because it feels like work to look at the world compared to watching TV. Or you grow accustomed to seeing so much, you can't center your attention properly. If you were to watch TV actively, like the experience of playing a computer game, you may enhance visual skills and reflexes compared to passive viewing. But for many people, passive viewing diminishes visual or imagery skills; and it retards emotional processing by sabotaging the natural mind's eye bridge between thoughts and feelings.

- **Reading away emotions** is a special category for poor sleepers, because so many use books and other materials to relax before bedtime or at night to return to sleep. Reading is an efficient way to relax and recruit the *Wave*, but you must evaluate why you read. If you read one romance novel every other day, the content of your books must be processing your emotions. Instead of facing emotions, you learned to "read" them away.

- **Self-medicating emotions**, wherein you change how your body feels with an external substance, the most common of which are food and alcohol, but also other substances, from legal to illicit. Smoking cigarettes and marijuana are commonly used to diffuse, diminish, deny, or smother emotions. Although these individuals may or may not be aware of their efforts to eat, drink, or smoke away emotional pain or discomfort, they usually sense that the behavior makes them feel better or more comfortable.

- **Intensifying one emotion** to avoid other emotions. Individuals who focus too much energy on sexual or hostile feelings, as two best examples, attempt to block other emotional experiences. The former seek episodes of promiscuity, adultery, prostitution, or pornography; the latter use brawling, other violent acts, or aggressive behavior such as raging at family, friends, or coworkers. Very intense religious feelings, if consistently in excess, can be used to avoid other feelings. The intensity in any of these patterns takes on an addictive character, making someone susceptible to cults. In the early phases, individuals do not perceive a problem; and in later phases, even if they spot something out of balance, the behavior is too entrenched, so individuals cannot perceive how to stop it and may have no desire to stop it.

- **Somatizing emotions** in which emotions are mostly experienced as physical aches, soreness, or pain. These individuals manage their "emotions" with pain pills, prescribed or over-the-counter. Some "somatizers" require stronger dosing and become narcotic-dependent. Others seek illicit drugs. The pain is real and intense, but part of their undigested emotional pain causes or adds to the intensity. The transformation of emotional pain into physical pain makes for safer and easier communication: "I'm in pain, give me medicine." Although more than half of us somatize occasionally (for example, kids' tummy aches when faced with homework deadlines or adults' tension headaches on a bad work day), those who regularly somatize are fearful or terrified of their emotions. To reverse a chronic pattern of somatization requires the help of a psychotherapist specializing in this area or an alternative practitioner such as a massage or bodywork therapist.

- **Psychotherapizing your emotions** in which, unfortunately, you connected with an incompetent therapist, traditional or alternative, who lets you talk and talk about emotions without engaging you to feel or process them, which is why the term "talk therapy" is an outdated, misleading, and ill-advised choice of words when seeking a therapist. This problem arises among individuals who report being in regular therapy for years or decades. When asked to describe what they learned or what specific skills they gained to strengthen emotional health outside of therapy sessions, many cannot respond with details.

> Trauma survivors are at high risk for receiving prolonged, inadequate, and harmful therapies because surprisingly, only a small proportion of therapists receive training to use the array of well-documented, evidence-based techniques for posttraumatic stress disorder (PTSD).

- **Medicating your emotions** in which a prescribing physician offers psychotropic drugs as the only means to manage emotional turmoil, without suggesting or recommending a credible form of psychotherapy to learn how to feel and work through emotions. A highly skilled and competent prescribing physician clearly explains that medication use is temporary or that a referral is necessary to a competent and trusted therapist to work with while on the medication. Unequivocally, the goal will be stated that therapy is designed to discover essential tools to strengthen your mental health, because medication is not always a reliable, long-term solution for many patients.

- **Talking** excessively for what seems like appropriate conversation, but that usually reflects an inability to monitor one's thoughts, feelings, and images. The person lives in a verbal world that permits the opportunity to release or burn up feelings with large quantities of speech. Such individuals can use racing thoughts at night to burn up anxiety, but it takes too long to be of much use. Extroverts are an exception to this style; they thrive in more communal or social lifestyles and can talk a lot while processing feelings simultaneously.

- **Fantasizing** excessively, in which great energy is used in the imagery world to live out one's emotions in narcissistic daydreams. These individuals develop some balance in the *TFI System* within their fantasies, because they are willing to use all three components in the mind's eye. Many fantasies try to resolve important emotional experiences or conflicts that the individual does not yet know how to resolve in the real world. If the person is rehearsing through fantasy for a real-world performance, imagery is useful and healthy. But when fantasies take on a life of their own, have no basis in reality, or are done in excess, they are clear attempts to avoid facing one's real feelings. Many artists or other artistic individuals learn to channel imaginative tendencies into art, which sometimes but not always reflects healthy forms of emotional processing. Many who fantasize in excess suffer shyness, another strategy to avoid emotions.

- **Channeling emotions** into socially acceptable activities such as work, religion, business, school, politics, athletics, hobbies, exercise, community service, or other volunteer activities. These approaches are some of the healthiest ways to work through one's feelings if you are unable or unwilling to work with them directly. All of us find that doing is an essential way to get through a particularly difficult time in our lives. This behavioral pattern should not be underestimated for its value nor deprecated as an inappropriate escape, because life throws lots of fastballs, curveballs, and a fair number of changeups. However, if the pattern is practiced to excess, it could also divert you from attending to your feelings, which may reflect some insecurity.

  > Politics is a noteworthy example. Individuals become so passionate about their views, they move their emotional turmoil to a place outside themselves. In bitterly contested elections, these individuals are on the verge of losing or downgrading friendships with those who don't share similar political views, which suggests that their emotions are running high for reasons beyond their civic duty. In the aftermath of close elections, unhealthy emotional investments in politics show up long after the votes were counted, with telltale signs:

  > > If on the winning end, the person continues to gloat and experiences an extremely inflated sense of relief.

  > > If on the losing end, the person continues to feel a sense of alienation, isolation, or perhaps an exaggerated sense of victimization.

- **Drowning emotions with more emotions** is a difficult style to understand. Individuals feel so many emotions so frequently or urgently, these feelings overwhelm them, making it difficult to sort out details about their most important emotions. These individuals are called "histrionic" or "hysterical," but a better term used by Dr. Leslie Greenberg of Toronto is "underregulators." With little regulation, emotions emerge all at once and all the time. This frequent display of emotion can be used to avoid feeling more specific or more painful feelings, but these individuals may be genetically programmed to feel and react more than others. Their goals in learning emotional processing skills are different from those of most people. We do not see this patient type in sleep medicine as often as others listed; but some trauma survivors suffer specific episodes of emotional underregulation.

The great irony in these descriptions is that emotions are truly designed to protect you, yet many of these behavioral patterns are clearly employed to "protect" you from your feelings and emotions.

Pattern Recognition

If you did not identify a pattern in yourself, it might be worthwhile to discuss these ideas with a skilled therapist, because the descriptions above are broad brushstrokes. The field of mental health has many other ways to categorize systems or styles for avoiding or weakly processing emotions, which could be important to consider.

Some but not all patterns described could be used in moderation for healthy emotional processing. A good meal or movie makes you feel good. A glass of wine or a beer relaxes you. A fun game of soccer or basketball produces a pleasant sense of tiredness. Nothing compares to making love with someone you love. However, when certain patterns are used excessively, perhaps you are not spending direct time processing emotions, which makes it nearly impossible to process vexing emotions.

With the aid of Little Big Step 9, determine whether you engage in a pattern or patterns of excess to avoid spending quality time with emotions. There is no recommendation or expectation now to change this pattern, but it is worth knowing whether these styles affect your sleep problems by preventing you from closing out the day or recruiting the *Wave*.

The most important question is whether you appreciate the concept of emotional processing. If you were angry, would you quickly search for the *Emotional Intel* delivered with the feeling, then work directly with this information to let the feeling come and go? Or when angry, do you eat, drink, play sports, work yourself silly, commit crimes, have sex, take pills, take drugs, think-think-think, see a doctor or a therapist, or feel lots of aches and pains in your body to the point of needing pain pills?

If you do not directly identify, feel, and then work through angry feelings, you might select from the menu above and, knowingly or not, engage in an alternate behavior to deal with these intense emotions. You can get very good at using these behaviors to deal with or seemingly wash away feelings. It can become a habit or learned behavior, in which you know no other way to tap into and process anger. In many real-life circumstances these styles prove reasonable, useful, and fitting for what's going on in your life at the time.

But not all the time!

Many of the pathways described are wastelands for your emotions. And if you reach the state in your life where, at bedtime, you cannot close out the day and cannot recruit the *Wave*, then you need look no farther than how you manage your emotions to identify the source of your persisting sleep problems. Curiously, there was a time very early in your life when you were supremely talented at emotional processing.

A Baby's Brilliance

Infants have the perfect emotional processing system.

- They are hungry, so they . . . cry.
- They are thirsty, so they . . . cry.
- They are in pain, so they . . . cry.
- They are uncomfortable, so they . . . cry.
- They are lonely, so they . . . cry.
- They are angry, sad, or afraid, so they . . . cry.

You could not invent a more ingenious, resourceful, reliable, effective, and beautiful system. Please notice how well these emotions ensure a baby's safety, survival, and well-being.

Unequivocally, the baby's emotions serve and protect him or her!

The baby experiences a wet diaper, an empty stomach, a dry mouth, a hostile environment, an unpleasant temperature, or the absence of love and immediately feels a strong emotion, then seconds or nanoseconds later, the baby processes the feeling by crying. What's particularly interesting is whether the baby's needs *need* to be met for a complete resolution of the problem, or whether crying itself resolves it satisfactorily. Babies need to cry when they bump their knees against a crib rail. The best fix, which a baby fully understands, is to wail; then the baby returns to a quiet state, as if nothing occurred.

Adults marvel at this process. It is phenomenal because it is so parsimonious. The baby quickly becomes aware of a feeling, then feels it, and then works through it as necessary, which lets it come and go. Instead of fighting with feelings and emotions, babies and most young children manage emotions by attending to them. Usually even strong feelings come and go.

This lesson should never be lost on adults learning emotional processing skills. For some troubled sleepers, you really need to start "acting like children."

Many other experiences in life, notably grief and bereavement, evoke emotions of a deeper intensity and duration that must be experienced differently. But the majority of emotional experiences on a day-to-day basis can be transformed into useful, information-gathering episodes (*Emotional Intel*). This process requires far less than a single day or hour; it's typically a matter of minutes or seconds, once you embrace the process.

When you work with your emotions directly, you prevent feelings and emotions from festering and corrupting your *Wave of Sleepiness*. Then you experience the *Day Is Done* in a natural and normal way. To arrive at this new place in which the feeling component of the *TFI System* is acknowledged and used throughout the day, you must stop fighting with your feelings.

Testing Your Emotional Intelligence

Before troubled sleepers learn to enhance emotional processing skills, they must determine whether they suffer misconceptions about emotions. It takes some work to identify and discard old ideas about emotions. Have you taken a SOLO moment to reflect on human emotions? Do you believe or recognize:

- that the purpose of emotions is to serve and protect you?
- what value or lack of value you attach to your emotions?
- misconceptions built into your views about feelings?

Most troubled sleepers who stuff or ignore feelings (arguably the most common style among insomnia patients) develop opinions that lead them to think emotions are useless or destructive. Some are so removed from their emotions, they cannot offer any opinion on what they believe about their "feeling system."

When you go through the following list of twenty-one true/false questions, answer them to the best of your ability by circling T for things clearly or mostly true or F for things clearly or mostly false. No doubt, you or others will debate some answers here, but the main objective is to start you thinking about your current opinions on human emotion.

Human Emotions Quiz

1. T F Emotions are mental things without a physical component.
2. T F Emotions usually take you back to old wounds from the past, making it difficult to work on current emotions in the present.

3. T F Emotions frequently betray you, providing information that hurts your feelings and makes you feel worse about yourself.

4. T F Complex emotions that generate anxiety and depressive disorders are best treated exclusively with medication.

5. T F Emotional problems cause mental health disorders, so working with emotions is too risky.

6. T F "Worry" and "stress" are more practical and useful terms to describe negative or unpleasant emotions.

7. T F Once you feel a strong negative or unpleasant emotion, it usually lasts a long time.

8. T F Feeling a feeling means the same thing as expressing a feeling.

9. T F Feeling your feelings is a sign of weakness or a character flaw.

10. T F Many emotions are too painful to be of any value or meaning.

11. T F Emotions are inflexible, lacking fluidity, which means they rarely change or transform into something else or some other emotions.

12. T F Spending time with your emotions leads to a touchy-feely personality, which leads to unproductive and worthless behaviors.

13. T F Working with emotions is disorganized and chaotic and will not organize or order your life in useful or productive ways.

14. T F Feeling a feeling feels like a loss of control, which leads to feeling overwhelmed or feeling like you are drowning in emotion.

15. T F Because it takes years to develop emotional processing skills, no immediate sleep benefits are gained by working with feelings today.

16. T F Learning to work with feelings will change a person for the worse.

17. T F Attending to your feelings will cause you to lose your sense of humor and make you too serious.

18. T F Spending time with emotions dredges up so many more emotions that medication will be needed to settle down troublesome feelings.

19. T F Learning emotional processing will not provide any benefits to someone suffering from an anxiety disorder.

20. T F Learning emotional processing will not provide any benefits to someone suffering from a depressive disorder.

21. T F Learning emotional processing will not provide any benefits to someone suffering from PTSD.

SLEEP ON IT
Evaluating the Quiz

QUESTION: How did you respond to the quiz?

COMMENT: Believe it or not, all the answers are "false" among individuals with healthy emotional processing skills. There are exceptions to every rule, and individuals with mental health disorders may discover some truth in a few scenarios on distinct occasions.

To be clear, working with emotions is not without potential side effects; and everyone is hereby warned that if your appetite to learn emotional processing skills is too large for your stomach, major indigestion can occur with the steps ahead. Nonetheless, debating these answers is less a priority than engaging in a frank discussion about how you see and know your emotions, especially how you do or do not feel them. Still, items marked "true" may be true for you.

Generally these statements reflect common misconceptions about emotions that are frequently propagated from generation to generation and in some cases from therapists to patients, with the patient often serving as a willing accomplice to the therapist.

SPECIAL RESOURCE: Sleep Dynamic Therapy coaches you on "sleep-related emotional processing skills," akin to the work of Dr. Leslie Greenberg in Toronto, who has spent years working and researching in the field of "emotion-focused therapy." For more general applications of these ideas, I strongly recommend Dr. Greenberg and colleagues' works, which include many outstanding, well-written books and research papers on emotion-focused therapy.

———— PEARL ————
Lay Your Emotions to Rest by Uncovering
Myths and Beliefs

To get the most from the quiz, let's reevaluate some questions.
First, note the items marked true; then spend a few minutes

reflecting on these ideas. Picture yourself in a situation in which these issues arise; then, if your reflection changes your opinion, change your answer for that question.

For items that remain, use a separate sheet of paper to jot down the full statement, or copy it elsewhere. Spend the next few days sorting out answers in real time. If you thought the first question was true, then the next time you notice an emotion, make the effort to determine whether it's only a mental thing or whether you feel something physical in your body. If you thought the eleventh question was true, the next time you feel an emotion, notice whether it really is inflexible or whether it changes into another feeling.

For pertinent questions, use SOLO moments to try to understand the responses you marked "true." If resources are available and you are comfortable proceeding, find a family member, trusted friend, clergyperson, therapist, or doctor to engage in a discussion about human emotions. Start by asking how they manage their feelings. Ask some questions from the quiz, perhaps focusing on the responses you marked "true." Gain some new ideas and opinions about handling human emotions.

The objective is not about definitive answers. Gray answers are what to expect in your discussions with other individuals, which lets you hear and consider new perspectives. If you get lucky and discuss emotions with someone with excellent emotional processing skills, that person would mostly agree that answers to quiz items should be false or mostly false in most situations.

In the upcoming chapters, we discuss various misconceptions presented in the quiz to explore how to improve your emotional processing skills. Without these skills, closure on the day and the *Wave of Sleepiness* remain out of sight.

16

Emotional Layer Cakes

Feel about It

Emotions come in all sizes and shapes . . . all flavors and scents . . . and all colors and shades.

To enhance your ability to work with them, please use the three-step sequence of identifying, feeling, and processing feelings. It's a lot like blowing up a balloon. The difficult thing is mustering the energy to expand the first part of the balloon, which is similar to early struggles and frustrations with pinpointing exact feelings or feeling something in your body. Once the balloon is partially inflated, your effort goes more smoothly, similar to what happens once you name a feeling or feel a feeling.

The dicey part of blowing up balloons is at the end, where blowing too hard pops it. In emotional processing, you may "explode" when you do not grasp how to process feelings clearly. However, as with balloons, you rest your hand on the back part to feel the tension (a feeling), which indicates when to stop blowing. While processing your feelings, you learn to see and feel the end point as well. In most situations, end points arrive without special effort, just like subtle but precise changes you feel in your breathing at full balloon inflation.

Let's imagine two examples of emotional processing needs. As we discuss these in the pages ahead, we'll focus on the second one, about work relationships, but the same applies to personal relationships:

- Someone in a primary relationship (spouse, partner, child, or parent) hurts your feelings, irritates, annoys, angers you.
- Someone at work (supervisor, colleague, coworker, or assistant) hurts your feelings, irritates, annoys, angers you.

When frustrated, how do you identify, feel, and process this feeling?

Many poor sleepers do not deal directly with this problem; they complain about it to someone else, especially in the workplace, which may or may not clarify the *Emotional Intel.* Most people talk about their frustrations to someone other than the offending individual because of anxiety about other emotions that might crop up:

- fear of losing a job if the offender has influence or authority;
- anxiety about an emotional backlash from the offender;
- embarrassment about having to confront the offender.

Checking Assumptions

Do you spot the fallacy in these three emotional reactions?

The *Emotional Intel* sounds negative or unpleasant, which certainly could be true in a blunt discussion with the offender. But this perspective begs the question because it assumes that the only or the best way to complete emotional processing is by talking with this person.

Emotional processing bulletin: *Absolutely nothing dictates that you discuss emotions with another person to resolve your frustrations.*

Instead, you must discuss your feelings with another and very special person in your life.

Namely, yourself!

To have a healthy discussion with yourself, please identify or name the feeling; don't call it stress or worry, call it what it really is: frustration, or perhaps anger. Next, permit yourself to feel frustration in your body, as discussed in the *Sleep on It* section in chapter 9; it generates tightness or tenseness in your chest, arms, hands, neck, back, buttocks, pelvis, legs, or feet. Using a SOLO moment, you are guaranteed to feel frustration somewhere, but you must stop doing and start being for a few seconds.

Then an amazing thing often occurs: the feeling will come and go. Nothing more was needed. You identified the feeling, felt the feeling, and by permitting yourself to be aware of your body, processing took care of itself. These three steps can take as little as ten seconds or less.

How so? Because the only thing needed, in so many more instances than most people imagine, was to just register the feeling itself . . . and not all the worries and ill-begotten thoughts you might have believed you needed to attach to the frustration or perhaps learned to attach to these frustrated feelings.

Now stop and reread the last few lines. You must understand how excessive thinking mucks up this process now and forevermore:

- By thinking about frustration, you cannot feel it.
- By not feeling frustration, you cannot let it go.
- By not letting it go, frustration drives you to think more.
- The cycle persists until it explodes with racing thoughts at night.

Unquestionably, when you process your emotions directly, you diminish racing thoughts, your mind-body slows down, and the *Wave* is welcomed ashore.

Evolving Emotional Intel

Frustration will not always come and go so rapidly. The feeling must be felt longer, or more processing is needed. The longer a feeling persists after someone frustrates you, the more likely the original emotion seeks to transform into a new and different feeling. When this change occurs, you want to watch for new *Emotional Intel* sure to arise from the new feeling. Here are five common examples of new emotions that might arise following a frustrating interaction at work:

1. *anger* because this may be a recurring experience of frustration that clearly interferes with your productivity at work;
2. *sadness* because you are not in a position to make your case to the offender;
3. *embarrassment* because you realize you are overreacting to a situation;
4. *forgiveness* because you appreciate that the offender did not intend to frustrate you;
5. *laughter* because you possess an appreciation for the imperfections of humanity.

The *Intel* in these five examples may permit relatively rapid closure of the experience if you feel the new feeling, then register and accept what it means. All the effort was accomplished within yourself. Only the anger or perhaps sadness indicates the possible need for action outside yourself, as part of your emotional processing. Then again, discretion may be the better part of valor, and no action need be taken right away.

Whatever the transformation, you must never forget this principle: Once frustration turns to anger or any other feeling, absolutely nothing dictates that the new feeling could not also come and go.

The Harmony of the TFI System

When you permit angry feelings into your body, you are blessed if you let new thoughts and images also enter into the picture, by letting the full *TFI System* capture essential *Emotional Intel* from the experience. A balanced *TFI System* reassures you in the midst of healthy emotional processing, and it feels very different than a bunch of worries and ill-begotten thoughts raining down on you. When a torrent of racing thoughts and ruminations throws your *TFI System* out of balance, it means you are trying *to fix the feeling instead of listening to it*. You also want your mind-body to recognize the emotion as part of a balanced system, so it anticipates and welcomes new thoughts and images delivering more *Intel*. When the three components of this system work well together to process emotion-based information, it feels like a three-part harmony—instead of a three-ring circus.

If your anger comes and goes, anger may be less intense than you first noted, but the issue that provoked the anger may still be relevant and in need of action or discussion. If your subsequent discussion with the offender occurs without anger fueling you to fever pitch, the conversation has a greater chance of finding a mutual understanding, if not an apology.

Threat Matrix

Sometimes anger proves most intense. What would you do if this feeling intensified and the balloon felt like it might pop?

When patients express this concern, I always ask, "How long does Old Faithful gush its strongest tower of water in Yellowstone National Park?" Most people who never visited the geyser respond that it must last five to ten minutes; a few say thirty to sixty minutes. In fact, the average time for Old Faithful to maintain its peak intensity is measured in seconds, almost always less than a minute.

The lesson is simple: intense anger frequently comes and goes more rapidly than you would imagine, even though you predict anger has a much longer half-life. The reason why anger can come and go so quickly is that it will often transform into another emotion. In more than 90 percent of instances, anger functions as a threat monitoring system, warning you of something that might interfere with what you are trying to do or be. Anger is a flare in the sky. It rarely offers complete *Emotional Intel*, but you have to receive the threat signal to move on to the next emotions containing the comprehensive *Intel*.

Insomnia patients are often affected by the vexing emotions of frustration and anger, but they commonly do not spot the flare and therefore do not see what's happening on the ground—that is, in their hearts. By not feeling, they do not uncover the next layer of emotion. They *think* about feelings, prolonging their shelf life, permitting them to fester and corrupt the *Sleepiness Wave* night after night.

Real Time, Real Layers, Real Emotions

The key to all these examples of processing is to permit your emotional experience to occur in real time, which quickly demonstrates how emotions are layered. Instead of waiting an hour, a day, a week, or a month to recognize an emotional response to something, now you recognize it while it's happening or soon thereafter.

With highly advanced emotional processing skills, little or no time lags between an inciting encounter and your ability to identify and feel a component of the feeling, regardless of when you process the feeling. This description is not about reactive or volatile people who fly off the handle. Such an individual is an "underregulator" and may not be capable of working with the full *TFI System* without professional help. With a balanced *TFI System*, you learn to travel through multiple layers of emotions in seconds. This potential might seem farfetched, but the capacity for instantaneous identification and sensing of feelings is natural, whereas delaying this process is a learned and relatively unnatural behavior.

Here's an example of moving rapidly through layers:

- A coworker forgot a task needed for you to finish your part of an assignment.
    You sense a feeling emerging, starting as frustration, because you wanted to complete your work today.
- Maintaining awareness of your body, frustration turns to anger, because the *Intel* reminds you that your coworker let you down twice before in similar ways.

By not fighting the anger, it comes and goes, preparing you to evaluate the threat.

Now you more accurately feel embarrassment or anxiety about your boss questioning your productivity, which leads to three interesting possibilities:

- If you are a weak emotional processor, you stopped before this layer, because you hate feelings of embarrassment or anxiety, so the anger sticks to keep the real *Intel* hidden.

  You fight with emotions the rest of the day, turning feelings into emotional bedbugs that take a large bite out of your sleep.

- If you are strengthening your emotional processing skills, you notice feelings of embarrassment or anxiety but find yourself perplexed about what to do next.

  You seem stuck, but spotting emotional layers is a big step forward. All emotional processing does not need immediate attention, so you may be able to sleep because there is less fear of emotions, which can be worked on . . . tomorrow.

- If you are a healthy emotional processor, you feel anxiety or embarrassment and let them transform into other emotions, or you know that your strong feelings dictate the need for a heart-to-heart talk with your coworker or boss.

  You go to bed with a clear conscience. Feelings may linger at low levels, but most of the intensity was processed as you rapidly pictured the real problem and scheduled a meeting.

Feel about It . . . Again

Going through layers does not require focusing on mental thoughts. If you come at anger from a "mental" viewpoint, you are still thinking your way through, not really feeling your way through. When you feel your way, it comes directly from your heart. The *Intel* comes faster and clearer, sometimes as imagery, which is how an episode can unfold and close itself out so rapidly. This entire processing sequence could take less than five minutes to clearly feel and then see what steps are needed. As your skill increases, this sequence takes less than a minute, including richly felt emotions coupled with crystal-clear *Intel*. The end result in the last example—the meeting—might occur right away or later. However, if the meeting was delayed, your clarity about the situation prevents the original, triggering feelings from infecting the rest of your day or your sleep at night.

If you believe you would waste a lot of your thoughts or other mental energy worrying about the upcoming meeting, please consider two possibilities:

- You may need a lot more development work on your emotional processing skills, but the good news is that you more easily recognize the imbalance in your *TFI System*.
- You may be deceiving yourself about what you accomplished the first time. Perhaps you really thought your way through with limited access to feelings.

When people use weak emotional processing systems, which are epidemic in business environments and workplace situations, *Emotional Intel* is ignored because feelings are ignored. This style drags the entire scenario across the office playing field for weeks, months, and sometimes years, which leads to grudges, ill will, and poor work performance. This soap opera is rarely worth an Emmy.

Revisiting Control

If you remain uncertain about developing your skills, spend a SOLO moment noticing the control you gain over your emotions by working directly with them. You no longer fight your feelings all day long, so they don't rise up at bedtime, activating your mind-body when you lie down to sleep. Emotional awareness becomes a natural part of your *TFI System*. When a feeling arises, you name it, feel it, acquire it (determine its *Emotional Intel*) and then process it (work out how and when to process the *Intel* and the feeling that inspired it).

Perhaps you are puzzled by your capacity to let feelings come and go. How can you turn red with anger and then let the feeling subside? To answer this question, consider the opposite one. What do you currently do now to process anger?

Most problematic sleepers ignore or stuff anger, creating some other fiction to control it. If they acknowledge it, it is usually in the mind only, which then sparks racing thoughts and ruminations. Few realize the "flare in the sky" concept and the essential *Intel* waiting to be scooped "off the ground." The next thing you know, the feeling part of the process was hijacked by your thinking component. The feeling festers inside your body, where it takes up space (rent-free)—in your clenched hands or jaw, your tight chest or stomach, or your stiff neck and shoulders. You lose awareness of these feelings in your body over time and do not connect how these emotions become physical symptoms. Ultimately you operate exclusively in your mind, so the feeling might get named at some point, but it never gets felt or processed.

If this closed system describes how you deal with anger, you can appreciate how difficult it would be for this emotion to come and go. In your shoes, since the emotion never really arrived, it cannot really depart, or as Dr. Greenberg frequently writes, "you must arrive at your destination, before you can leave from there." What can we do at this point to help you arrive at your destination, to that place where you permit yourself to feel a feeling and not reflexively "think" it into oblivion? The answer to this question may be much easier to relate to than you might imagine, because undoubtedly you are already engaging in this behavior for most if not all of your happy or pleasant emotions.

Little Big Step 10: Happiness Is a Great Teacher

Take a moment to be sure you know how to identify, feel, and process those feelings in your life we all describe as positive or pleasant:

- happiness;
- joy;
- contentedness;
- relief;
- satisfaction.

The ideal way to start is to complete the three-step sequence of identifying, feeling, and processing the feeling from memory, based on a recent experience from today or yesterday. Start with a SOLO moment, then picture something that made you feel good. Once you are clear about the memory, spend time using imagery skills to reexperience it. See yourself go through it a few times. Then go back into the memory and see yourself:

- identifying or becoming aware of the feeling in your mind;
- feeling the feeling and becoming aware of it in your body;
- processing the feeling to see how or what makes it come and go.

We accept that happiness does not last forever. In these exercises, you want to see how this process takes you up temporarily, but more importantly when the happy feeling has gone, notice how it should not leave you down or empty. Your feeling state or mood might be relaxed or neutral or nothing special, but you would not expect to feel unhappy; you would not expect the loss of happiness to turn your mood sour.

Once you conduct this imagery exercise on a three-step processing of a memorable positive feeling, then test it in real time. For the next few days, make a special effort at least once per day to notice how a positive or pleasant feeling courses through your body, stays awhile, and then leaves. The *Emotional Intel* offered with pleasant feelings are some of the most memorable and enjoyable experiences in your life. Be sure to use a SOLO moment to kvell these feelings (a Yiddish term for relishing, especially relishing your kids). Last, notice how pleasant emotions last only a few seconds or minutes; then the feelings leave your body.

Also, you may notice that a strong, positive feeling like happiness or joy that triggers ruminations could also block the *Sleepiness Wave* at night. This valuable lesson teaches you that it is emotions—strong feelings in your body—that corrupt the *Wave*, because these physical feelings taint the feelings of sleepiness. Although this idea seems obvious, you may discover that by sensing corruption from pleasant emotions, you may reduce your nervousness about resolving the corruption from unpleasant emotions.

Why? Because you learn that feelings are sometimes just that—physical sensations in your body, whether positive or negative, that are more than capable of coming and going.

If you get stuck working with positive emotions, do not frustrate yourself. This step should be relatively easy for most, but if not, ignore the suggested emotions above and focus strictly on laughter—that is, identify, feel, and process the experience of laughing at a good joke or some other funny thing.

Therapeutic Laughter

An insomniac sees a doctor about his sleep problem. "Doc, every time I get into bed, I think there's somebody under it. But when I get under the bed, then I think somebody's on top of it. Top, under, top, under . . . all night long, I'm going crazy!"

The shrink says, "Come three times a week for two years and I'll cure your fears."

"How much do you charge?"

"A hundred dollars a visit."

The insomniac hesitates. "Let me sleep on it."

Six months later the doctor runs into the guy on the street. "You never came back to see me," bemoaned the psychiatrist.

"For a hundred dollars a visit?! A bartender cured me for ten bucks."

"What'd he say?"

"Cut off the legs of the bed!"

Assuming you have not heard the joke, it usually generates a smile or a chuckle. If you have ever been in therapy, you might laugh out loud. The question at hand is, "What are you experiencing in the act of reacting to [smiling, chuckling, laughing at] this joke?"

The answer is that you are engaging in an abbreviated but highly advanced and instantaneous form of emotional processing. Responding to the joke is a shorthand version of emotional processing, because you don't have to do anything to identify or become aware of a feeling. You also don't work to feel something in your body, because when you smile, chuckle, or laugh, each change in your face, throat, or chest represents a change in feeling in your body. Last, you don't work on processing feelings, because the fact that the joke induced you to smile, chuckle, or laugh indicates that you processed the *Emotional Intel* by laughing.

There are two jokes. The first occurs halfway through the story in which an insomniac desperate for help reflexively says, "Let me sleep on it." This joke pokes fun at him in the same way we laugh at a man repeatedly trying to drink water from a glass with a hole in the bottom.

In the second joke, more germane to troubled sleepers who've been in therapy, we discover that common sense (the bartender's advice) is as powerful and clearly less expensive than a trained professional's advice. The joke pokes fun at a lack of common sense among therapists. The more you laugh at this second joke indicates that you have had or know of encounters with therapists who did not possess much common sense. Your laughter permits the opportunity to release (process) instantaneously whatever feelings you registered from past dealings with therapists. Laughing them away is a form of pure emotional processing, which requires little thought. The entire process is induced by the joke.

Please don't confuse this discussion with an overanalysis of a simple joke. Humor proves to be one of the most advanced forms of communication, if not specific therapy, because it carries a big punch, yet the punch never hurts unless it splits your sides. Humor can provide instantaneous emotional processing even if you have no patience or interest in working on your emotions or the time to do it.

Silver Bullets

When helping certain individuals detached from their feelings, we start their emotional processing efforts by working only with humor and laughter. The original *I Love Lucy* episodes with Lucille Ball and Desi Arnaz are a common suggestion, as are the Three Stooges, Laurel and Hardy, and numerous other television or movie actors and characters. I prescribe one dose of laugh-out-loud video or movie viewing per day.

When you use laughter to feel more, make mental or written notes about what occurs. Here are some questions to consider: When you laugh, what do you feel in your throat, face, chest, stomach, arms, or legs? When you're done laughing, what do you notice afterward about your breathing, the tension in your hands, shoulders, or neck, your self-talk, the way you feel, the pictures in your mind's eye, and especially the way you communicate with the first person you find yourself in contact with?

Nothing in your quest for emotional well-being is as important as your sense of humor and your capacity to laugh. Among people who develop mental health disorders, the loss or drying up of one's sense of humor is one of the earliest signs of an impending problem. This is truly serious business, because taking oneself too seriously causes mental health problems or worsens mental health symptoms. You must be able to laugh, and to laugh at yourself.

If you appreciate this wisdom, consider humor and laughter as the best starting point when you have difficulty feeling your feelings. Through humor you can receive the immediate bonus of improvements in mental health and sometimes improve your sleep as well by learning to laugh again and learning to laugh at yourself.

Although sleep problems are no laughing matter, our objective is to teach you how to engage the feeling component of the *TFI System*. Laughter is potent medicine in the development of your emotional processing skills. Sometimes you find yourself laughing so hard you cry, which is another advanced technique to shed some tears over.

Therapeutic Tears

With laughter, you may never identify any particular feeling, but you feel something in your body. Crying often proves as powerful as or more so than laughter, and like laughter, you cry over happy and sad things. You may never precisely identify the feeling that provokes tears, but you feel something in your body, including the feeling of tearing up or tears pouring out like rain. Afterward you processed some emotion, even if you cannot explain things.

When you laugh or cry, you release emotion embedded within you, whose name is no more precise than physical tension. The crying or laughter breaks up the tension and releases its hold on your body. You feel something powerful coursing through your body when you belly-laugh or cry like a baby.

You may feel clueless about the cause of this strong reaction, which seems like an exaggeration, given you may never know why you laughed so hard or cried at all. After this emotional release, your body feels similar to how you feel after making love. You'll notice less self-talk, greater imagery in your mind's eye, and a more relaxed and comfortable feeling.

To use crying techniques, dig out memories from the attic. Life is bittersweet, so there's a lot to choose from. Your greatest stumbling block could be the belief that crying is a sign of weakness or a character flaw, even if you cry in complete privacy. If these barriers thwart you, consider whether you learned these beliefs for reasons that no longer serve you.

Most people benefit from a good cry. But if you feel worse afterward, you should only work this way with a therapist. Among those coming to our sleep centers, more than 98 percent report benefits releasing emotional tension in this way.

Here are keys to help you:

- Find material from the past you know will make you cry, such as the closing scenes with Judy Garland in *The Wizard of Oz* ("There's no place like home") or Jimmy Stewart in *It's a Wonderful Life* ("A toast to the richest man in town," followed by "Auld Lang Syne"). Many movies bring you to tears.
- Consider crying whenever you feel strong emotions but cannot identify them, and you are confused about what to do with them.
- When you well up or tear up, notice if something inside stops your crying. Pay close attention to determine what blocks you.
- Usually you feel blockage in your facial muscles; they feel tense or your expression is contorted as you try to cry on one side of your face and try to hold it back on the other side. If tears are hiding, they usually burst forth when you let your facial muscles relax around the mouth, cheeks, or chin or even the throat area.

- If you struggle to cry, consider help from a family member. Some people feel shame crying alone but are capable of crying with someone they trust. You might attain a deep cry with support from a therapist. Massage or bodywork therapists can help you release a "muscular dam" holding back tears.

After you complete a good cry, notice how:

- your neck, shoulders, and chest feel more relaxed;
- you breathe easier and stand up straighter;
- racing thoughts diminish;
- imagery is more accessible;
- long your emotional well-being lasts.

Never underestimate the power of crying. One good cry per week markedly enhances the balance in the *TFI System*. Crying releases much emotional tension without necessarily going in depth through all the emotional processing steps. Although you want to work at higher levels of emotional precision, use a good cry to your advantage as a reasonable and excellent way to move toward that goal. Finally, next time you hear someone say "I almost lost it," now you know they almost lost their version of control over their emotions. However, after a healthy cry, you might find yourself one day declaring "I found it" when you discover heartfelt and invaluable *Intel* from your emotions.

Physicality

When you look carefully at instantaneous emotional processing techniques such as laughter, crying, or making love, it's easy to see how physical they are, and this pattern may mislead you into thinking that other physical things yield the same results. You may wonder whether running, jogging, walking, or swimming all produce the same ends. Regular physical activity is good for sleep health and provides some emotional processing. Brisk walks clear the head. But don't confuse exercise with advanced emotional processing obtained from laughing, crying, or sex. Physical actions burn off low-grade tensions, such as some anxieties or frustrations, and the physical actions distract your mind as you use your body. As physical energy is burned, you feel relief of emotional tension, too. Or your mind percolates on emotional issues, uninterrupted by self-talk, during exercise.

In comparison, laughter, crying, or sex release much greater quantities of emotional energy than exercise, because they are so emotional. These instantaneous forms are like waving a magic emotional wand over your body. You don't gain a full understanding of how the process unfolded, but you become aware of successfully processed emotions. Instantaneous emotional processing techniques should be used by everyone but are most important to those who fear learning too much from their emotions. These techniques are potent enough to release emotion and recruit the *Wave of Sleepiness* in rapid fashion.

SLEEP ON IT
Express Yourself to Yourself

QUESTION: The greatest confusion in working with your feelings arises when a person believes that feeling your feelings is the same as expressing your feelings. Concern arises that once an emotion emerges, it must be expressed to someone else. So let's ask: How much do you express your feelings to other individuals?

COMMENT: Most people experience 99 percent or more of their feelings without expressing them to anyone. Yet emotional awareness is blocked by a belief that you must share your feelings with others. The best example is the emotion of anger, which most people imagine is directly linked to aggression. To feel anger means to act aggressively, so it is wiser to stuff it. But channeling anger into aggression almost always develops as a learned behavior. Anger is a powerful feeling that courses through your body; you feel hot; you might look red; but the amazing thing is that nothing in life's rule book dictates acting on the anger. Sometimes you should act, but more times you can feel anger without expressing it to anyone but yourself.

This self-expression of emotion is the key to your emotional development, because it gives you license to feel your feelings, whatever they are. Self-expression neither precludes taking action when appropriate nor forces action when inappropriate. As logical as self-expression sounds, many individuals fear the feeling of anger. Usually these fears are based on two themes, which you must consider when stuck developing your emotional processing skills:

- Fear of *Intel*: You fear an emotion because it only dredges up other feelings, thoughts, and images that make you feel worse.

- Fear of fear: You fear feeling an emotion because its *physical feelings* in your body feel unpleasant, like a loss of control, or like you are drowning in emotion.

These beliefs may bear some truth. If you don't like the fear-induced adrenaline rush on the down ramp of a roller coaster, you would not seek to feel this fear. If you notice that your anger makes you more irritable with family, you would not see any value in feeling angry.

─────── PEARL ───────
Develop a Taste for Emotions without Causing Indigestion

The key to feeling feelings is to know what it means to really feel a feeling. In your experiments with happy or positive feelings or with laughter or crying, you want to feel something decidedly physical, regardless of the meaning you attach to these sensations. Certain emotions produce strong physical sensations that feel overwhelming, such as the heat of anger, the depths of sorrow, or paralyzing fear. But few people live a life of this intensity every hour of wakefulness, every day of the year, or even every week of the month.

Most of us have little to fear from these physical sensations, but when you ignore emotions, they feel uncomfortable, unusual, or strange. This strangeness becomes habitual and blocks all efforts to explore feelings. Your task is to observe how your values, beliefs, judgments, insights, opinions, and reactions color emotional experiences and stifle emerging *Emotional Intel*.

Weather offers an excellent metaphor. The feelings of heat and cold or wetness and dryness produce feelings in your body, open to different interpretations. Wetness of rain coupled with thickness in the air could produce melancholy if you were living a single lifestyle, but it could also intensify romantic feelings if you were falling in love. Physical sensations of wetness and thickness are present in both situations, but you perceive or appreciate these sensations in different ways based on circumstances.

If you appreciate the physiological side of emotions, all your work on emotional processing goes smoother. Besides, you already "taste" many physical aspects of feelings and emotions throughout the day:

- needing to use the bathroom;
- tasting and feeling your food being chewed and swallowed;
- putting on your clothes;
- anticipating the day ahead;
- joking with friends;
- working intensely with colleagues;
- playing with your kids or helping them with homework.

All these experiences generate feelings and many emotions. You may not pay much attention to these feelings, but they are there, waiting to be explored, valued, and acted on. Surely, most appreciate the *Intel* "gotta go, gotta go" from your bladder. So why not learn to view more of your emotions in this way and learn to receive them when first delivered?

By starting with simpler areas of feelings and emotions, you can retrain yourself in preparation for working with deeper, more intense emotions. By learning to feel all your emotions with great precision, you can prevent them from tainting your *Sleepiness Wave*.

If you get stuck anywhere in your efforts, you must take a deep breath and honestly ask yourself whether you believe that "human emotions serve and protect you." If you are not ready to accept this principle, then by all means consider working with a therapist, or review the sections on laughter and crying and stay with these approaches until you make some breakthroughs on your perspectives about human emotion.

17

Feel the Feeling, Then See It Clearly

Pure Emotion

When you are not afraid of your feelings and permit yourself to feel them without adding in all kinds of worries, ill-begotten thoughts, or perverse judgments, then clear and genuine *Emotional Intel* emerges.

When you explore *Intel* using all components of your *TFI System*, the emotion usually diminishes in intensity. You act appropriately, because you did not fight with or pile onto your initial "pure" feeling. Without this sequence of behaviors you are likely to shoot from the hip. Here are four examples of working wisely or weakly to manage a pure feeling:

- While dancing, you step on your partner's toes, provoking embarrassment with which you could laugh at yourself and apologize, or quickly shove the blame onto your dance partner, believing that shaming him or her will relieve your feelings.
- Someone cuts in front of you in line for a movie ticket, provoking anger with which you could speak your mind, then forgive and forget, or start a heated confrontation with the other moviegoer and be on the receiving end of the first punch.
- Your VCR or DVD player won't play the movie, provoking frustration with which you could take a deep breath and reassess the situation, or show the inanimate object who's boss and pound it with your fist.

- You swerve preventing an accident with a reckless driver, provoking *fear* or *rage*, which makes you pull off the road safely and thank heaven you're still breathing, or put the pedal to the metal, taking your life right into someone else's hands.

Choose Wisely

Why would someone choose the first set of healthy emotional responses versus the second set of ill-advised responses?

When you are embarrassed, you may believe or know you hate this feeling, because it makes you feel small, vulnerable, or self-conscious. Since you hate it, you would rather pass it off to someone else. Yet embarrassment is only trying to say you are human—nothing more—you made a simple mistake. Perhaps you could ask for help from your dance partner to avoid this misstep. Instead of receiving the *Intel*, you worry about your embarrassment, which leads you to feel more embarrassed, turning it into shame.

Make no mistake about it: you learned this self-defeating behavior.

When angry, you may not like the feeling of being threatened—anger's alter ego. If you hate this feeling because it makes you feel powerless, then it's no surprise you might overreact to demonstrate power. Yet anger is only telling you that a threat is present. You must analyze the situation with your *TFI System* to determine whether the threat is high or low, real or imaginary. Someone butting in line is a low if not an imaginary threat.

Again, you learned this self-defeating behavior.

When frustrated, you feel incompetent or inadequate because you cannot stand that something made of plastic thwarts your desire to be entertained. Yet frustration only shows you that something isn't working properly. Perhaps you need to more carefully work through the steps to connect the movie-playing device. Maybe you need to reread the instructions. There is a reason why all electrical appliance troubleshooting manuals begin: "Please check that the power cord is plugged into the electrical socket." If you respond to frustration with impatience, you are ignoring the *Intel* and will respond in ways that make you imagine you are "stressed out."

Again, you learned this self-defeating behavior.

When fearful, perhaps you were scared out of your wits because you thought the end was near, or you were enraged by someone driving so recklessly. These strong emotions activate your mind-body to a state of high alert to ward off a dangerous threat. In fact, you averted danger; you swerved;

thus your system worked perfectly. The incident is over, but once your mind-body gears up for survival mode, it takes time to cool down. If you remain unaware of the way your body works, you could take up the chase and drive yourself down a dangerous road.

These and many other learned behaviors routinely interfere with your ability to recruit the *Wave* night after night.

Little Big Step 11:
Counting Your Emotions

The previous scenarios provide typical day-to-day examples of how someone learns to work ineffectively with emotions, and these patterns provide food to the emotional bedbugs taking a bite out of your sleep. Now we need to get down to the business of spotting exactly how feelings corrupt your *Wave*, so you can prevent this corruption from happening.

Frustration and anger are the two most common emotions that fester day to day in the body to corrupt the *Wave* at bedtime or at night. Spend two days taking stock of these feelings in various situations:

- Count them up.
- Make mental or written notes about what provoked frustrated or angry feelings.
- Notice how quickly you sense these feelings emerging in each situation.
- Pay special attention if you find yourself in situations that should provoke frustration or anger, but you do not feel these feelings.

Today's work is for realizing how often in a single day "things go against the grain." You may want something, need something, are trying to do something, and some barrier stands in the way. This conflict produces a feeling: frequently frustration, occasionally anger. The first phase of the exercise is to see how many times in a single day you are exposed to this stressful situation. By the way, if the only way you know how to perceive these frustrations is by labeling them "stressful," please do so for now. However, stress is not a precise feeling, which therefore can mislead you. More on this point shortly.

After a day or so of counting, spend a few days observing. You should now possess a greater capacity to observe your mind-body, using the SOLO skill to know:

- what frustration feels like;
- where you feel it;
- if it moves to other parts of your body;
- what thoughts and images emerge during the feeling;
- how long the feeling lasts;
- what makes the feeling go away.

Last, if you have trouble letting go of the feeling, try to observe what makes the feeling stick like glue. The SOLO technique is especially helpful when used as a neutral observer. Pretend you are conducting an experiment to learn about human emotion; your goal is to observe feelings in your own mind-body to learn what the experience feels like. Your objective is neither to attach judgments to your emotions nor to analyze them to death. You wish to observe this experience in a reflective and unbiased manner so you feel emotion without doing anything about it just yet.

Most troubled sleepers spot many more episodes of frustration and anger in the course of a day than previously imagined. Just by counting and observing them, a problematic sleeper grasps how the daytime gives birth to emotions crying out for attention at night.

The Gatekeeper

At this point, the single greatest barrier to your success in counting and observing the corrupting influences of emotions comes from your choice of words to describe emotional experiences. For example, in the last step you may have discovered that you don't usually notice feelings of frustration or anger. Instead, you frequently use the terms "stress," "worry," "anxiety," or "depression" to talk about emotions. If so, you may not know how these terms block you from feeling your feelings and how they prevent you from processing them. How could these words be so powerful?

Several factors play into this problem:

- These words reflect real and painful conditions, but these terms are too broad and prevent you from naming precise emotions.

    The more you use these terms, the farther you move from precise feelings, and your understanding of specific emotions may fade away.
- By accepting these terms as the only explanation for emotional turmoil, the TV commercials and culture that inundate you with this

viewpoint lead you to believe that medication is the only way to process human emotion.

Although psychotropic medications work wonders in some, many patients state that these medicines numb their emotions, diminishing their ability to feel feelings and gain *Emotional Intel* from them.

- When you grow accustomed to these words as the best or the only way to describe emotional turmoil, your use of these terms prevents you from appreciating clearer emotions.

All these terms function as gatekeepers that block out precise or clear descriptions of your feelings.

When you become habituated to saying "I'm stressed out" or "I'm depressed," you lose the capacity to reflect more precisely on your emotional state, and you lose out on *Emotional Intel*. In so doing, you rarely see that more precise emotions almost always fuel the very conditions we often label as stress, worry, anxiety, or depression. Overcoming this problem is not easy. Just observe what happens in the workplace and in other social gatherings. A substantial proportion of people with emotional difficulties constantly bemoan their current lifestyle or circumstances:

- "I'm so stressed
- . . . or depressed
- . . . or worried
- . . . or anxious!"

If you asked these people what they meant by any of these expressions, they would look at you as if you landed from Mars. If you pushed it more, you would provoke someone into experiencing a clearer emotion, such as anger or fear, which they might be clueless on how to process.

On the other hand, if a close friend or family member were open to real dialogue, you quickly get to the heart of the matter—that is, extremely precise emotions in response to extremely precise experiences frequently underlie use of gatekeeper terms. With some discussion it would be clear that depression might be due to a long-standing neglect of a series of precise emotions. As an example, the person might have had a great deal of anger, frustration, and sadness brewing about a work problem over many months or years that was never identified, experienced, and processed and thus eventually transformed into depression.

Many qualified psychotherapists know the process described above and are up in arms about so many afflicted individuals receiving only a pill to solve a problem that took years to develop. Competent therapists recognize that pills may help but do not *cure* the problem called "depression" in most people who try pills, because pills do not directly target the lack of attention to the emotional layering affecting most depressed patients.

The medications cure perhaps a quarter of patients who use them and make improvements in as much as another 50 percent, so their benefit is beyond dispute, but it does not appear that emotional processing skills are routinely offered with the prescription, which sets up many patients for relapse and limits their capacity for further mental health gains.

Identifying Your Gatekeepers

The perspective described above is absolutely critical to hear if you wish to pursue sleep-related emotional processing, particularly if you believe you cannot sleep because you suffer from "stress," "worries," "depression," or "anxiety." You may suffer from these conditions, and you should consult with your doctor or therapist on how to treat them. But it is also critical to your sleep to change the way you describe your emotions, because your descriptions restrict or expand how you learn to work with feelings. To prevent feelings from tainting your *Wave*, I am not recommending changes in medications, psychotherapy, or other pathways; rather, emotional processing should supplement your current experience.

One of the first rules offered to problematic sleepers, particularly those who believe that "stress, anxiety, worry, and depression" prevent them from falling asleep or staying asleep, is to red-flag these terms. Whenever they use or hear one of these terms, the first thing to consider is whether they are hiding from precise emotions or they don't know how to uncover them.

Using these broad terms as a starting point to discuss your feelings is fine and may prove beneficial. However, if you remain fixated on these terms—for reasons unrelated to an actual diagnosis of a mental health disorder such as major depression—then you must learn to appreciate: **you are not engaged in an effort to identify, feel, and process precise emotions.**

A traffic line lengthens, a light turns red, a cashier speaks rudely, your kids bicker, your boss demands, you forgot the umbrella, you burn dinner, and the beat goes on in the course of real life; something unexpected, undesirable, or unpleasant occurs in the midst of ten other things you happen to be juggling in the modern hurry-and-worry world.

How do these things really make you feel?

In the postmodern world, people use the term "stress" to describe these experiences. Why is "stress" often an empty, useless, and deceptive term to express feelings? Because when you default to a communication style in which stress is the catchall for all your emotions, you have just handed yourself the *Reader's Digest* version of how you really feel.

SLEEP ON IT
A Mind's-Eye Feel for Feelings

QUESTION: As your emotional processing skills increase, you want to integrate them with your imagery skills. Imagery bridges the gap between thoughts and feelings. When you think or feel too much, imagery can restore the balance in your *TFI System* by moving you away from racing thoughts or extreme feelings. Have you applied imagery skills to connect your thoughts and feelings, and have you used imagery to clarify your feelings?

COMMENT: Your visual system, of which your mind's-eye imagery is an integral component, has tremendous capacity to engage, organize, and re-create daily events in your life. Take an episode of playing with kids. If you embrace the experience as a special thing, the visual feast makes up the best part of your experience. You delight in their playfulness, mischievousness, smiles, affection, and genuineness. Your eyes help to organize activities, monitor potential problems, maintain safety, and promote camaraderie. At a later time, you re-create the experience in your mind's eye.

All three of these processes—engaging, organizing, and re-creating—are natural parts of your visual/imagery systems. If you were to "think" your way through, it would turn into a flat story, whereas your eyes make it a 3-D adventure. The eyes have it!

The visual and mind's-eye images predominate because a picture tells a thousand words. The feelings and thoughts linked to the pictures in front of you or your mind's eye are just right because you engaged the experience with your eyes. Please consider this point for many daily tasks in which you may not engage your eyes much. Think about certain work situations or a situation with your kids where they need to complete homework. Do you use your eyes as much as you could? Or is your brain grinding with too much thought or your body grinding with excess tension? The following Pearl offers a better way.

——— PEARL ———
The Pebble-in-the Pond Imagery Tool

Your imagery system works in many situations to produce a more satisfactory outcome, yet this skill is often underutilized or not even discussed with:

- parents to help them raise kids;
- mental health patients to help them overcome their distress;
- sleep patients to help them sleep;
- employees to help them be more productive and satisfied.

How do you advance this skill to bridge your thoughts and feelings? The first great secret to imagery is its 24/7 availability. The second secret is that you can tap into it in seemingly fanciful ways, yet gain rich insight. Reflect a moment on a recent problem. Do not select a big one; pick something minor. This exercise is different from when you changed something in your mind's eye. Changing the furniture did not reflect a problem or the need to change the furniture.

You would like a degree of conflict that you seek to resolve. If you had a recent minor problem in which you were angry at someone, use that example to learn about processing anger. Many other experiences suit this exercise, ones as simple as trouble finding your car keys. Once you select it, retrace a number of thoughts and feelings on this issue for just a minute or two to remind yourself of recent memories about it.

Follow the next steps in the comfort, privacy, and safety of your home. You need ten to twenty minutes for the whole practice, although many discover that five minutes are sufficient. Once skilled in this technique, a minute is adequate. First perform pleasant imagery for a few minutes to activate the system positively. Then open your eyes and reconfirm in your mind or verbally the nature of the minor issue. In other words, be clear about the problem.

Now close your eyes and picture a pebble dropped into a pond of water. Once the pebble hits the water, see the water rippling outward. Here's the most powerful step: avoid engaging too much self-talk; just picture the ripples of water, because if you see ripples, new images usually pop into your mind's eye. These images are often new insights to solve the problem.

The images may provide a clear picture that offers an obvious solution; or they may spur you to change or transform your original feelings or reconfigure your thoughts. When a new idea or thought emerges, it does not feel like the usual self-talk or chatter; it possesses more clarity and a feeling of value, like a "lightbulb" effect. There is nothing hokey about this skill or about the capacity of your brain to function in this way. Your brain has the knack to solve problems rapidly using imagery, similar to bringing up a map in your mind's eye to give directions.

Use this skill now to test this process. Try it in as many circumstances as you can. Notice how thoughts and feelings were previously unable to solve the issue, but imagery bridged these TFI components to lead to a solution or new directions. Once you are skilled in the pebble-in-the-pond exercise and obtain good results, you can generate new images without visiting the pond. Soon you appreciate that a picture forms in your mind's eye whenever you experience feelings, conflicts, or other problem-solving or troubleshooting situations. The picture might be right before your eyes in an encounter that provokes feelings. Or the picture emerges in your mind's eye. These images prove extraordinarily helpful in finding instantaneous balance during intense situations, which pushed you toward too much thinking or feeling.

Please make a concerted effort to notice the invaluable relationships among your feelings and your thoughts and the images in your mind's eye. As you advance, consider this question: Can you change your feelings or your thoughts by changing the images in your mind's eye? The answer is unequivocally yes, but you may need more practice with your imagery skills.

18

Clear Sailing through Cloudy Skies

Return of the Gatekeeper

When you look inside the window to your soul, is it clear or cloudy?

Emotional clarity is a hallmark of people who permit themselves to feel their feelings. When you are clear about emotions, you easily identify them and feel a clear feeling in your body, after which processing is natural. Because the *Emotional Intel* is extremely clear as well, in most circumstances processing occurs quickly or definitively.

The greatest barrier to this clarity arises with the misconception that emotions are somehow static or stagnant experiences. Instead of operating as a fluid and flexible part of your *TFI System*, emotions feel a lot stickier if not unchangeable. Once you start feeling a feeling, you may fear it's going to last forever and lead to a breakdown or a meltdown. The misconception that feelings have no end or do not transform into something else leads many astray in their quest for emotional clarity.

From the previous discussion on "stress," "worry," "anxiety," and "depression," it is critical to recognize how these global terms persuade you to think that little can be done to change how you feel. When you pursue stress management classes or take medications, they may help; but if they do not enhance emotional processing skills, these therapies may fail you in time.

To gain emotional clarity, you must see how cloudy emotional experiences actually prevent you from seeing clearly on the inside. The most common form of cloudiness is produced by gatekeepers, which prevent you from feeling clear feelings.

The Worry Warpath

One of the best examples of the gatekeeper is worry. Worry is frequently used to ward off or cover up deeper, precise feelings, which you were afraid of or uncomfortable with. A game of hide-and-seek is sparked by worry, eating up more time and energy, as if you could wait out your emotions. Here's a complex yet common example of how a worry gatekeeper blinds you.

Financial stress produces racing thoughts, which turn to worries about something that:

- has occurred—you must pay off past credit card debts;
- is occurring—your checkbook balance must meet present needs;
- will occur—your future debts will soon be incurred.

When problematic sleepers report racing thoughts about finances at bedtime and blame this behavior for sleeplessness, they miss an important part of the equation driving sleeplessness—the emotions that drive the racing thoughts. After all, in the dead of night, how much will your:

- checkbook worries grow your account balance by morning?
- finance charges decrease by stewing over credit card debts?
- rate of return go up stressing about long-term investments?

As you know, these mental calculations about dollars and sense might just as easily contribute to your financial health as make your financial misery index soar. Perhaps you solve some financial issues at night, generating useful ideas to increase income or decrease expenses. Few are so lucky. Most spin their wheels about financial pressures with worry-filled, racing thoughts. Yet few poor sleepers engaged in the worry mode identify the building blocks of worry. It's not the self-talk, negative ideas, or stress that infect your body with physical tension. These cloudy elements aggravate worries, but rarely are they the driving forces.

Clearing the Path

Clearer emotions are at the heart of the matter:

- You fear going into debt; thus fear provokes worry.
- You are angry you didn't get a raise; thus anger provokes worry.

- You are disappointed you couldn't afford a gift for your child; thus disappointment provokes worry.
- You are frustrated by the rising prices of gasoline, heating fuel, and medical costs; thus frustration provokes worry.
- You are embarrassed or ashamed that you can't take your family on a nice vacation; thus embarrassment or shame provokes worry.

Each feeling may come in isolation or as a group when experiencing financial concerns. Each one brings critical *Emotional Intel*, providing highly specific information you almost never spot when stuck in a pattern of worry-stress-worry-stress. These specific emotions send clear messages if you have the courage to listen to your heart:

- Your *fear* may be saying that you must consider a second job to solve the current crisis.
- Your *anger* may be saying that your employer is untrustworthy, which means you must rethink your career potential at this job.
- Your *disappointment* may be saying that you have overemphasized material things in your relationship with your child.
- Your *frustration* may be saying that it's time for a fresh look at your budget.
- Your *embarrassment* or *shame* may be saying that it's time to review your priorities and ambitions.

Make no mistake about it: *Emotional Intel* provides these instant messages if you listen for them, but if you choose a worry warpath, you do not discover what's eating you up inside.

Many troubled sleepers, confused about the purpose and value of emotions, learned to worry about or focus on stress, which is like thinking all the way around the borders of a swimming pool instead of jumping in for a swim. All of us fear the water will feel too cold, be too deep, or cause a shock to our system, so we continue to speculate (worry) about what swimming feels like instead of actually swimming. The more we engage in worrying or reflexively labeling our worries as stressful, then the real clear, primary emotions fester, intensify, and eventually feel so powerful that once you jump or get shoved in the water, you feel a sense of drowning momentarily.

Your worry gatekeeper blocks deeper, clearer, more valuable emotions from your awareness due to your discomfort with these feelings or your fear of their *Intel*. Ironically, ignoring clear feelings generates more cloudy feelings of worry. You've made your bed but can't sleep in it!

Truth Be Told

Financial worries mirror the problem of troubled sleepers' weak attempts to process emotions. All day long, primary feelings go unprocessed; people register the experience as "I'm stressed," "I'm depressed," "I'm worried," or "I'm anxious." After a long day, they do not change this view; rather they move to another indirect form of emotional processing, such as drinking alcohol, watching TV, or talking with friends and family but not about emotional events and rarely about precise feelings. Real clear feelings continuously fester and intensify; then bedtime arrives, brain waves speed up, the mind-body is restless, and inevitably:

- The *Wave of Sleepiness* is far out to sea.
- The *Day Is Not Done.*
- *You really do not want to be asleep.*

Having ignored emotions all day, something must pop up at bedtime, in the middle of the night, or in the early morning, and that something is an unprocessed emotion in the form of:

- racing thoughts and ruminations if you tend to think too much;
- anxious or tense feelings if you don't see layers in emotions;
- unpleasant images if you avoid developing your mind's eye.

Now you are ruled by all these elements, because each one produces significant closure problems that cause at least an hour's delay in falling asleep, another hour or two of middle-of-the-night awakenings, or another hour lost by cutting your sleep short.

The best approach to this problem is to work with your emotions during the day, because technically **insomnia starts first thing in the morning, right when you get up**—as soon as you start stopping emotions from coming into view. Over time you can learn new skills to apply throughout the day, and these steps are the best long-term approach to emotional processing and to insomnia as well.

Little Big Step 12A: Where to Start

In the heat of the night when the worry demons come out to frolic, what plan of action can we develop to turn the tide in your favor so you peacefully continue your sleep quest? This step is the longest one and is divided into four parts, but it will show you how to sleep when emotions run too high.

When swords are drawn at bedtime or in the middle of the night as the battle to sleep or not to sleep unfolds, your first task is to measure how far the *Wave* is from shore. Using the SOLO tool, notice whether you are sleepy and assess the frequency of your racing thoughts or worries. Then you need to transform any thoughts or worries into precise feelings, so these emotions can come and go, to welcome the *Wave* ashore. However, before proceeding, you must decide where you want to work on these steps.

The prudent advice is to get out of bed. Bear in mind that once you learn these skills, your comfort level will permit you to achieve your goal in five to ten minutes. You will be able to complete this sequence, then go to sleep. For now it's best to work on this step away from the bedroom. Start by reviewing a few racing thoughts or worries, and look for a pattern or a theme to describe the content racing across your mental landscape. Within these thoughts, careful scrutiny will identify something bugging you, often about relationships, money, responsibilities, or tasks needing time and energy. Spot a pattern or a repeating item.

For this example, you notice you are spending time thinking about a relationship with your kids, spouse, parent, grandparent, or perhaps a friend or a coworker. You notice that your mind keeps replaying something that's happened. You also want to notice whether some feelings emerge. The most likely feelings would be of discomfort or anxiety. You feel ill at ease about what's occurred between you and the other person. This process takes several seconds or several minutes. Many problematic sleepers struggle here, because they cannot make the leap from racing thoughts to a feeling of discomfort or anxiety.

If stuck, use the SOLO technique and review key body parts to see if you find the feeling hiding. Key places to explore include:

- Mouth, teeth, jaw, or hands: are they clenched?
- Shoulders and neck: are they sore, uncomfortable, or tense?
- Chest and sides: is your breathing slightly restricted?
- Stomach: is it queasy or tied up in knots?
- Back: is it achy or painful?
- Legs: are they restless?

You may believe other explanations for these physical feelings. But if you are stuck, it is worthwhile to consider that the emotion you cannot link to racing thoughts has found a home elsewhere in your body. A sure sign validating this connection would be a change in the feeling in your body, one way or the other. The feeling lessens because you permitted yourself to feel the emotion you are clenching in your teeth, or it worsens as your stiff neck holds back the emotion. Either change confirms the presence of the emotion in your body.

Little Big Step 12B: Turn a Thought into a Feeling

In attempting this part of the twelfth Little Big Step, you often discover emotions wanting to escape to deeper hiding places. You may feel more physical aches, pains, and tension if prone to a somatizing style of processing. You may only be capable of finishing the rest of this step with a therapist, massage therapist, or other bodywork specialist. Assuming you locate a feeling, let's assume your first impression is discomfort, but nothing more precise.

Harness your imagery skills to complete the next step. Quickly review the self-talk that led to your awareness of an unresolved relationship issue. Try to connect the self-talk to this discomfort. If stuck, picture you and the other person for several seconds and ask yourself "What am I uncomfortable about?"

At this point expect another change; the most obvious one would be that the feeling isn't just discomfort, it's more specific: anxiety. You recognize anxiety about this relationship, although you are not sure why. If you feel anxiety, you deserve kudos as you transformed racing thoughts into a feeling. If you feel anxiety—truly feeling it in your body, not thinking about it in your mind—you discover a decrease in racing thoughts. This change means you are moving in the right direction.

Anxiety as a Mischief-Maker

If anxiety produces more racing thoughts, consider whether you are struggling with feeling your feelings. The self-talk reemerges at a faster clip, along with anxiety, to take back control, because you hate the feeling of anxiety. Now the content of your self-talk fills up with more unpleasant judgments, criticisms, and sarcasms, heaped on top of anxiety. Again, you learned this style to prevent yourself from reaching the depths of your feelings; worse, this negative self-chatter can send you toward an emotional brink. If so, you may need professional help to overcome your self-destructive use of the *TFI System*.

Little Big Step 12C: Let It Come and Go

Assuming you have awareness of anxiety, and the self-talk has diminished slightly, the next phase creates three possibilities:

1. Anxiety comes and goes on its own; nothing more need be done. Usually racing thoughts have markedly diminished, leaving the *Wave* in plain view.
2. Anxiety doesn't exactly leave, yet by feeling it for a while, a useful mental recognition occurs about this relationship issue and the need to explore it—say, tomorrow. Such an expectation is satisfying enough to let the *Wave* approach.
3. Anxiety transforms into another emotion—let's say anger—which then either:
   - comes and goes on its own;
   - comes and stays until you gain more *Emotional Intel*, which transforms anger into another feeling, which then comes and goes;
   - comes and the *Emotional Intel* is completely processed or you gain confidence in knowing how to process it later, which resolves the anger or quiets it down.

In the last three experiences, the *Wave* gains sufficient strength to lap upon the shore.

Now let's examine the three transformations from anxiety to anger listed in example 3. To reach the anger, the troubled sleeper often must talk herself there. If she feels anxiety yet it doesn't transform quickly, she must talk herself through it, as follows: "Right now I'm feeling anxiety, which is a gatekeeper feeling often used to cover up another feeling; therefore, what is the most likely feeling I'm covering up?"

Then picture the relationship in your mind. If you cannot feel the feeling yet, you can usually identify it as something like, "Oh, yes, the most likely feeling is 'fill in the blank.'" Or, in this case, "Yes, I am probably feeling anger." Once stated, you will feel it somewhere in your body, perhaps one of the key body parts described above, even if it's as simple as a change in your breathing to deeper or shallower breaths, or the rate of breathing slows or quickens. Emotions have strong physical components, which are easy to spot once you become accustomed to observing your body.

Assuming you felt a physical degree of anger, this single discovery may completely connect all the dots and prove sufficient unto itself, as in "Yes, that's what's bugging me about the relationship. Now I have it in my sights. That's all I needed to know, thank you very much."

What if anger is stickier? More *Emotional Intel* may need uncovering. You might stay with the anger for a couple of minutes and let it emerge gradually. The *Intel* might cause the anger to transform again into another emotion such as fear, sadness, guilt, or embarrassment, which brings more *Intel*. And by allowing yourself to feel one of these clearer feelings, you receive *Intel* much faster, after which the new emotion may come and go.

The pebble-in-the-pond exercise described in chapter 17's *Sleep on It* as well as the one later in this chapter may be most useful when you are closing in on *Intel* but not quite there yet.

Little Big Step 12D: Wave Good-bye to Insomnia

Let's say you are now ready or close to ready to get back into bed.

In the scenarios above, the *Wave* is close, and for some it sweeps onto shore, putting you to sleep in no time at all. In fact, sometimes you fall asleep so fast after an emotional processing experience, you forget what it was about or how it happened. The reason for this delightfully forgettable experience is that the *Wave* was never far from shore. As soon as it saw an opening, it swept in to carry you to Nod.

To summarize, let's restate the opposite of effective emotional process-ing to emphasize the power of cloudy emotions: the anger you were hold-ing on to—in the disguised form of anxiety—was preventing you from finding closure on the day by generating racing thoughts and an undercur-rent of cloudy emotional tension and worry that continuously corrupted your *Wave of Sleepiness*.

Recognition and resolution of this process put you to sleep in no time at all. Make no mistake about the possibilities of gaining immediate relief through initial use of your emotional processing skills, even though you will work on your skills for years to come.

Most troubled sleepers can learn to complete such an exercise in less than ten minutes the first time they try it. But over time and practice, you can rapidly put two and two together in a few minutes or seconds, especially when you have embraced the idea that balancing your *TFI System* is an extraordinarily healthy way to view things.

Summary of Bedtime Emotional Processing Steps

Please review these steps any time you are stuck with an unpleasant emotional experience at bedtime or during the night:

1. At bedtime, you notice racing thoughts.
2. Using knowledge linking racing thoughts to a disguised emotion or a mental activity designed to avoid emotion, you exclaim, "I have racing thoughts; I'm hiding a feeling."
3. Recruiting the *TFI System*, select a technique to identify the feeling as:
   - imagery to picture what feelings might be present;
   - feelings to directly feel something;
   - thoughts to predict what the feelings might be.
4. The most common tool is thinking in which you realize that anxiety, unease, tension, or another ill-defined feeling lurks beneath racing thoughts.
5. Having made a prediction, racing thoughts ease slightly, then you apply the knowledge that anxiety is a cloudy emotion or gatekeeper.
6. Again, recruit the *TFI System* to feel the anxiety as:
   - discomfort in your chest or throat;
   - butterflies in your stomach;
   - tension in your arms or legs;
   - tightness in your hands.
7. As soon as you notice a feeling in your body, racing thoughts decrease because you shifted attention and energy from your mind and toward your body.
8. Next, if anxiety might be a gatekeeper, reflect on whether this feeling is linked to something to be anxious about, or whether anxiety is covering up another feeling that dropped off your radar screen earlier in the day.
9. Recruiting the *TFI System* again, use thoughts, imagery, or a sense about other feelings to clarify the true feeling provoking anxiety.
10. At last, something breaks through, which may be:
    - a thought: "I have a hunch it's anger."
    - a feeling: "My body is no longer feeling anxious, it's feeling something else with heat, fire, stronger breathing . . . like anger."
    - an image: "I recall an incident in my mind's eye from earlier in the day when someone slighted me, and I tried to shrug it off."

11. You link the emotion to earlier in the day; it started as irritation and grew to anger because the incident or irritation festered and intensified.

12. As racing thoughts are cut in half, if not more, a final step asks: How do you process this feeling of anger so it comes and goes?

This raises the question of whether you believe anger will come and go. If you believe it will, because geyser jets typically last for less than a minute, then feel the feeling, acquire the *Intel*, and watch the anger dissolve or convert into another feeling, with new *Intel*.

Never lose sight of how clear this pathway is compared to ignoring your emotions. It may take time to walk this walk, but when you grasp these steps and confidently apply these skills, the whole thing becomes its own SOLO minute—for many, a few SOLO seconds. Now you know that the real culprit is not racing thoughts, not worry, not anxiety, but a real clear feeling that you can process to let the *Wave of Sleepiness* rock you to sleep.

SLEEP ON IT
Sleeping Bedder and Bedder

QUESTION: An exciting thing about enhancing imagery and emotional skills is that most individuals can combine their work in these realms. Do you see yourself as someone who can connect your images and feelings, or do you worry they might overwhelm you?

COMMENT: Weather again teaches a lot about paying attention to sensations in your body. A sunny or a rainy day offers different pictures that stimulate various feelings in your body. You don't just feel melancholic or romantic on a rainy day, you also see the rainy day. You don't just feel hot or cheerful on a sunny day, you also see the sunny day.

Why is this concept so important? In almost every instance, a picture goes along with a feeling. The picture might be right in front of you as the encounter unfolds. Or you may replay this picture with the imagery in your mind when you find yourself revisiting the feeling.

Trauma survivors know this process well. For them, the difficulty arises when pictures in their minds never resolve but linger, provoking more bad feelings. These mental health patients must be cautious in working with imagery and emotions, but with professional therapy, they reap great rewards by learning to connect images and feelings, then processing them. Everyone operates in the realm of thoughts, feelings, and images. The question is whether you are comfortable moving yourself into a position to spend time with both feelings and images in an effort to balance your *TFI System*.

With recent exercises you used imagery to solve a minor problem in your life. Now our goal is to connect imagery and emotion. The last exercise in this chapter tackled the problem of bedtime anxiety. Our objective is to repeat that exercise with greater emphasis on imagery. After you practice, try it the next time you feel anxiety at bedtime.

———— P E A R L ————

Advanced Imagery Is the Ultimate Ticket to Dreamland

As with any imagery exercise, begin with a pleasant scene and stay with it for five minutes, letting images come and go. Then use the pebble-in-the-pond approach, but start anywhere you like in the anxiety scenario you have chosen to work with. For example, you could be suffering from racing thoughts, or it could be clear that you are suffering anxiety. Either problem is a red flag, signaling that some deeper, clearer emotion is hiding. But this time you will not go down the sequence of twelve steps to uncover the real clear feeling. Instead, shoot the moon and attempt to uncover the real clear feeling through the pictures in your mind.

You might still start with "I notice my mind is racing," or "I'm feeling tense or anxious," or "I am not sleepy when I think I should be." Then start the pebble-in-the-pond imagery while pondering one of these themes. Again, just have a theme in mind as you limit your self-talk. Your goal is letting images emerge from the ripples in the water.

Let's assume a similar example: some relationship in your life causing frustration or anger. What I am suggesting in this rerun of the exercise is that when you go directly from racing thoughts (thinking) or anxiety (feeling) to the pebble-in-the-pond imagery, you gain the potential to bypass all other steps. You just might go directly to the heart of the matter and find the precise emotional content as well as the precise emotional solution to the problem in less than a minute.

You must not confuse this instruction with rehearsing images over and over about a recent conflict. Use a more neutral starting point of ripples in the water: let images come up, and let images change. Many of our research patients with nightmares who learned imagery skills reported this exact process—that is, once they let images into their mind's eye, they discovered that imagery would change, as if seeking a solution or providing a series of options from which to choose.

The change in images or new images triggered a change in feelings, indicating the potential for immense power with imagery. Successful people in all walks of life use imagery regularly, including a skilled therapist who evokes a mind's-eye solution when managing a patient in crisis; a professional golfer bringing forth a mind's-eye solution to a critical golf shot; or an intuitive business executive who welcomes a mind's-eye solution to help the company progress.

The picture or pictures that spring from the mind's eye—when you are receptive to this imagery process—provide a wide array of *Intel*, which combines information derived from thoughts, feelings, and images. In other words, the mind's eye offers an instantaneously balanced *TFI System* at your beck and call. When you achieve this capacity to juggle effortlessly the full spectrum of thoughts, feelings, and images, you have reached a pinnacle in your development of your emotional processing skills.

Repeated use of the exercises in this chapter, with special emphasis on coordinating your developing imagery skills with thoughts and feelings, often brings you rapidly to a place in which you can use emotional processing skills to effectively eliminate insomnia on almost every night. It's an especially powerful tool for those sorts of nights for which you once felt so much exasperation.

You need only let the picture show begin!

PART FIVE

BIG TRANSITIONS TO SOUND SLEEP

Good-bye, Sleeping Pills; Hello, Missing Links

Turning Little Big Steps into Giant Steps Forward

All readers will benefit from concluding comments about emotional processing at the beginning of chapter 19, because the information will prove invaluable in learning to sleep without drugs and in learning to sleep in new physiological ways to promote high-quality slumber. Also, other transitional information, in chapters 19 and 20, is needed for certain readers.

In chapter 19, those who want to stop using sleeping pills are offered steps for tapering off use of such medications. All you've learned to this point proves essential in making this transition as smooth as possible. The more confidence you have gained in using imagery and emotional processing skills, the greater your chances for success.

In chapter 20 we discuss the transition from the mental to the physical treatment of sleep disorders. Skimming or reading carefully through this short chapter depends on your readiness to treat physical sleep problems.

19

Emotional Freedom to Sleep without Drugs

Emotions Always Win!

Emotional processing is easier to attempt and simpler to complete when you heed this challenging perspective: emotions always win!

Do not mistake this adage to mean that emotions rule you. Just the opposite; by staying vigilant to your clearest emotional responses, you remain in charge of redirecting your emotional experiences, based on the invaluable *Emotional Intel* you have unlimited access to. Because emotions always lurk beneath virtually all human experience, your efforts to observe emotions and work through them in a timely way prove an efficient and meaningful way to live your life. You will grow comfortable attending to your feelings and only rarely find yourself surprised or overwhelmed by them, mostly in special or unusual circumstances.

Emotions always win because feelings are designed to deliver their messages, but if you choose not to answer the doorbell, the message must be delivered in some other way, sometimes more urgently. You know the side-door approaches you adopted, such as worried thinking, headaches or backaches, stressing out, and so on. Countless examples describe the ways in which individuals transfer the delivery to another part of their *TFI System* except the one most capable of processing emotions: the feeling component.

Unprocessed emotions will win out and fuel insomnia because you really do not want to be asleep when unappreciated feelings demand your attention. In so many instances, your mental wheels are spinning out of control, yet these wheels need an engine. If you look under the hood, you discover that your body is feeling something, which provides the fuel to keep your wheels churning past bedtime and beyond. You would never worry unless unfinished emotional business caused you to worry. Emotions can drive the troubled sleeper to imagine that whatever was accomplished during the day was insufficient to draw the curtain on the day's performance.

Sooner or later you want to realize that if emotions push you to work the night shift, then you elected to work overtime. The irony is that you would never go to work intending to sleep, yet it appears you go to your place of sleep intending to work.

Emotions always win!

Still, you might not believe that worry or anxiety could be working to hide your deeper emotions. Many see these theories as idealistic or impractical approaches to how we manage our feelings. Emotional processing is not a panacea, but it is a valid, reliable, effective, and powerful tool for most individuals with sleep problems; and it is highly useful and necessary for those who have been led to believe that sleeping pills or other medicines are the best or only way to overcome troubling emotions at night. Nearly all such regular users of sleep medications became dependent on or habituated to these drugs in large part due to their inability to work effectively with their emotions.

On any given night, the goal is to help you get to sleep and stay asleep. When you engage in basic emotional processing during the daytime, very little emotional residue lingers at bedtime to prevent the *Wave of Sleepiness* from lapping gently on the shore all night. In time you will discover that sleep-related emotional processing is one of the most powerful tools to maintain in your sleep recovery toolbox.

Sleeping through It All

As you address these psychological components of *Poor Sleep Quality*, never lose sight that you are also repairing your broken sleep by decreasing physical sleep fragmentation. If you were successful in your efforts, then you have been slowing down your mind, body, and brain waves, all of which leads to *Sound Sleep*, the sleep you really need.

Now is the time to ask whether your medications—prescription, over-the-counter, or any other sleep aids or substances—are also decreasing your sleep fragmentation and enhancing your sleep quality. Certain patients benefit a great deal from medications, so continuing to use them may be the better option. To sort this out, it's useful to compare the impact of your medications versus the impact of Sleep Dynamic Therapy (SDT).

As you make comparisons, keep in mind some of the theories and controversies that support or reject the use of sleep medications for chronic sleep problems.

- Do you need sleep medications because your body is wired differently than normal sleepers'?
- Would psychological and/or physiological treatments of your sleep disorders eliminate the need for sedatives?
- To be sure, we must state categorically that benefits from medications may be dramatic for some patients. The question then is: Have they produced dramatic results for you?

Sleeping Pills or Not

A natural system supports sleep without medication. If you want to stop pills, it is more useful to demonstrate results from the natural system prescribed by this SDT program first, before making changes in the dosage or frequency of medicine prescribed for sleep. Many who have worked to this point have obtained good to excellent results and probably have discussed medication changes with their prescribing physician. Others who have been using over-the-counter remedies may have noticed initial tapering or elimination. For those still dependent on a medication after engaging in the SDT program, please be mindful of two potential influences:

1. A physiological sleep disorder persists in fragmenting your sleep, which prevents you from attaining an optimal response to the psychological phase of the SDT program. Your best bet is to conquer your physical sleep disturbances first, then taper your medication.
2. Your genetic predisposition or neurochemical markers in your brain may be imbalanced in ways more responsive to medication. Although this condition is rare in my opinion, it may require medication. A local sleep specialist may be your best option in sorting out this issue.

Little Big Step 13: Planning Stages to Stopping Pills

To stop using sedatives or other drugs for sleep, you must work through five principles:

- Establish if medication was ordered for sleep problems only.
  If not, clarify what you will do about other treatment needs if you stop the drug. Would you need another medication for anxiety or depression, or would emotional processing skills suffice?
- Clarify your biggest reasons for wanting to stop the medication.
  Side effects of sluggishness in the morning or memory disturbance during the day are common reasons, but the most common is that sleeping pills don't provide consistent sleep quality improvements or even sleep quantity improvements.
- Seek guidance and support to reduce or eliminate sleep meds.
  Most prescribing physicians are supportive in this area, but they may not have much experience to guide you through the tapering. The most valuable service they provide is to monitor for side effects and how to treat them urgently.
- Write down the name, dose, and use schedule of the sleep med.
  Visit the Internet for the specific drug you are using or discuss with your pharmacist or doctor to determine its half-life, which is a general measure of the time it takes to eliminate the largest amount of the drug from your body. A short half-life indicates a potential for a more rapid tapering, whereas a longer half-life indicates tapering for weeks or even months.
- Organize a tapering schedule of the drug with the assistance of your prescribing physician.
  Taper in ways least disturbing or frustrating to your sleep patterns. Some patients taper from a 10-mg dose of zolpidem through repeated 2.5-mg reductions every two weeks or so, such that two months were needed to stop the medication; but others cut the dose in half the first week, used 5 mg every other day the next week, and then used the drug once per week thereafter, or as needed for special circumstances.

Who's Been Sleeping in My Bed?

Unless you are suffering from a serious side effect or some other medical or psychiatric emergency, it is never advisable to stop taking sleep aids abruptly if you use them regularly. It is almost always advisable to follow the five principles outlined above. Stopping cold turkey typically worsens your sleep and produces more serious side effects than those caused by the sleep aids.

Among those severely dependent on a sleep aid, particularly alcohol or prescription medications, it is highly beneficial to your health, your well-being, and your sleep to address this issue only after you clearly made progress with other components of the SDT program, unless you are hospitalized or working closely with your doctor or therapist to taper off use of these substances.

I cannot emphasize this point enough, particularly among people who already recognize that they are dependent on a prescription medication and want to get off it. Now may be a fine time to taper off medication, but you absolutely must establish that you can use the new tools from your sleep recovery toolbox to supplant medication. You must feel reasonably confident in activating imagery skills, recruiting emotional processing skills, and in the heat of the battle, knowing it's okay to lose a little sleep as you go through the tapering process.

Timing is everything. And, as a barometer of your readiness, if you have conquered the time barrier, you have an excellent chance of tapering medication; whereas if you have yet to give up time monitoring and calculating, you should forgo trying to eliminate medication now.

SLEEP ON IT
Sleep Medication Tapering

QUESTION: It's remarkable how many troubled sleepers go off sleeping pills on their own. It may occur because they learned something else to help themselves sleep. But more often, they just became disgruntled with the sedative approach because it didn't work or it made them feel worse. Even so, a sizable proportion of those who use sleeping pills need to carefully check their concerns, motivations, and rationale to go drug-free before doing so. Have you made this assessment?

COMMENT: Mental health patients with problematic sleep show the greatest anxieties and fears when going off sleeping pills. Most of these individuals were led to believe for years or longer that prescription sedatives were the most reasonable way to approach insomnia. As mental health problems clearly worsen their sleep quality and quantity, it seems logical to stick with meds. And mental health patients require more time and coaching to change self-defeating learned behaviors, find closure on the day, and enhance sleep quality. If success has brought them to a place where the *Wave of Sleepiness* appears upon their shoreline, then their chances are much higher for successful tapering. Now they can recruit the *Wave* and expect sleep to arrive naturally.

Regardless of your progress, if you have important reasons to reduce or eliminate sleeping pills, a specific treatment known as sleep restriction therapy can be combined with your tapering schedule to get yourself over the hump. However, sleep restriction therapy is an emotionally anguishing approach to solving insomnia. I rarely offer or recommend it in severe cases until a patient has made sufficient progress in developing imagery skills and embracing emotional processing skills. These skills make sleep restriction less daunting, more tolerable, and more effective. Treating physical sleep disorders beforehand also makes things easier.

Sleep restriction therapy is based on the homeostatic principle that the less you sleep, the more you should feel sleepy. Your objective is to restrict your sleep with a singular motive: deprive yourself enough so you feel sleepy the next night. A classic example involves someone who spends eight hours in bed but sleeps only six hours. The instruction changes the schedule to decrease time in bed to only six hours—the amount equal to the total sleep currently obtained. This step puts a lot of pressure on insomnia patients because now they are thinking they have only six hours in bed to get six hours of sleep.

Although these instructions seem extreme at first, almost all who attempt sleep restriction notice within a couple of days and certainly within a week that they are feeling sleepier at bedtime from the sudden drop in hours of sleep at night. Usually the *Wave* returns in fairly pure form, the individual recognizes and welcomes back the pleasurable feeling of sleepiness, and in days, they report dramatic improvements in their ability to fall asleep. Moderate improvements in their ability to sustain sleep through the night occur as well.

In more severe cases—say, the individual who sleeps only two hours per night while spending eight hours in bed—the choices are scarier. It would be next to impossible to persuade yourself to spend only two hours in bed, because it would feel like self-inflicted torture. Such individuals, though can start by slowly reducing time in bed by an hour per week, and usually long before they arrive at five hours in bed, they see increases in sleep.

Any variation of sleep restriction therapy, be it decreasing the number of hours in bed or decreasing the actual number of hours slept via an alarm clock, can be combined with tapering of sedatives. Because sleeping pills may confound your perceptions of your natural *Wave of Sleepiness*, it is essential to ensure that you are clear that the *Wave* is nearby when use of sleeping pills is tapered.

Many sleep physicians tailor sleep restriction programs for those patients seeking to eliminate sedatives, and all use steps designed to work in parallel with the tapering schedule, such as those described in the following Pearl.

——— PEARL ———
Sleep Medication Tapering Guide

1. As best you can, adopt a sleep schedule for a week prior to tapering.
2. Keep track of hours slept and hours spent in bed.
3. For the week, take the average number of hours slept and divide by the average number of hours in bed.

    6 hours of sleep ÷ 8 hours in bed = 75 percent of the time spent asleep.

4. Raise this percentage (aka sleep efficiency) above 85 percent and preferably above 90 percent.

    As above, decreasing your time in bed to 7 hours yields 86 percent (6 ÷ 7) and is the fastest way to get started, but you may soon find total sleep time increases to 6½ hours, yielding 92 percent (6.5 ÷ 7).

5. Use this new schedule for about three to seven days and then start tapering.
6. Stick with one sleep restriction schedule for a week, but if you notice a worsening of insomnia, always tweak the sleep schedule before making further changes in medication. Tapering changes always come *after* a new change in the sleep schedule, not the reverse.
7. Taper along a comfortable plan, whether two weeks or eight weeks.

    Remember, you must know the half-life of the drug so your time frame is reasonable. Drugs such as lorazepam, alprazolam, and many antidepressants used for sleep require longer tapering than sedatives such as zolpidem.

8. You may need to tweak your sleep schedule up or down to accommodate your circumstances and comfort level, and sleep doctors are the ideal medical professionals to advise you in making these subtle changes.

9. Active use of imagery and emotional processing skills will consistently aid in overcoming difficulties in recruiting the *Wave* during the tapering.

10. Now might be one of your best opportunities to apply sleep hygiene instructions to help you support the new organized structure of your sleep schedule. A set wake-up time each morning can prove helpful.

11. Once you achieve your objective of reducing or tapering medication, maintain sleep restriction for several weeks to stabilize your efforts, then consider the potential value or risk in gradually increasing your number of hours in bed, if you perceive that more sleep is needed.

12. Never forget that a physical sleep disorder may underlie insomnia and poor sleep quality. If you stop medication but are not satisfied with the impact on sleep quality, commit to working step-by-step through the assessment and treatment instructions on physical sleep disorders, or visit a sleep center for the same. For many patients, treating the physical sleep disorder should precede any tapering.

20

Counting Blessings instead of Sheep

Bodying the Mind

Some sleepers reach this point and believe they have achieved all the gains they need, while others thirst for more. When we move to the next section, there will be those who imagine that physical sleep disorders just could not apply to their problems. And there will be those who imagine that the strategies learned in the earlier sections could not possibly carry over.

My sense is that most people who read parts six and seven will be in for a series of discoveries of such astonishing proportions that they are likely to run up the flag on the pole of skepticism faster than you can say "Sleep on it." Because sleep is so culturally steeped in ideas surrounding the mind and not the body, it is a huge shock to your thinking to discover that something physical is a major factor in your broken sleep.

Of further interest, you will learn how your emotions play a critical role in your ability to accept this new information and how to apply appropriate strategies to resolve physical sleep disorders. Most remarkably, you will hear a tantalizing theory of how emotions may actually cause physical sleep disorders.

You should be excited about knowing that all your development work on your imagery and emotional processing skills can turn out to be the greatest assets to help you overcome any barriers to successful physical sleep treatments. My goal has been to bring you to a place where you experience

Sound Sleep and the *Sound Mind* that emerges from healthy slumber. Many readers with a more pronounced psychological perspective on sleep believe they have already made sufficient gains and feel thoroughly satisfied.

I am here to honestly tell you, "You ain't seen nothin' yet."

Little Big Step 14: Consolidate, Consolidate, Consolidate

In your sleep recovery toolbox reside many precision tools you can use regularly to improve your sleep. Don't hesitate to review past sections, especially little big steps and pearls to keep your momentum going forward. Please pause here for a moment to realize that everything you have learned can be consolidated into one sentence, long though it may be:

Your mind and your body can monitor and then develop a balanced operating system based on a flexible and fluid flow of thoughts, feelings, emotions, and images, which stimulate richer and more satisfying daily experiences, culminating in a strong feeling of closure at the end of the day, which then triggers a powerful feeling of sleepiness and imaginative dreamlets to carry you to sleep and keep you there as long as needed; and by using your powers of observation to monitor the thoughts, feelings, emotions, and images within your mind and body, you can simultaneously learn to slow down your brain waves, balance your operating system, and develop the skills to rebalance it in difficult times.

At this point most have made significant gains in the following ways:

- taking less time to fall asleep at bedtime;
- fewer awakenings during the night;
- greater ease in returning to sleep if awakened;
- more solid hours of sleep each night;
- benefits from improved sleep quality, such as:
  - more energy;
  - less daytime sleepiness, tiredness, or fatigue;
  - sharper mental faculties;
  - more stable, relaxed, or happier mood.

Take some time now to reflect on what were the most important steps in helping you achieve these gains. What helped you turn things around? Make sure you know what worked for you and what might be worth trying in the future. You might wish to revisit some sleep hygiene instructions in chapter 6, which may seem easier to apply now. When you think back about any attempted strategies, notice how much easier they can be implemented as your *TFI System* is moving toward greater balance.

The following five sleep hygiene rules or related strategies are some of the most powerful tools at your disposal when properly applied. Were you able to use these tools?

1. Eliminate time-monitoring behavior.
2. Wake up each morning at the same time.
3. Sleep in a darkened bedroom.
4. Use your bed and bedroom only for sleep and making love.
5. Not lying awake in bed for long periods of time trying to sleep.

Give yourself a SOLO minute, reflect on your accomplishments, and let yourself feel positive, upbeat, and confident about what you achieved. Hang on to that confident feeling and teach yourself how to recall just how capable you can feel when you know how to solve a problem with your own mind and body. That's the spirit you want to take with you into the next section, because you want to use your *TFI System* every step of the way.

SLEEP ON IT
Physical Sleep Disturbance Keys

QUESTIONS: As we move to the physical side of sleep problems, you will be intrigued by an entirely different set of tools that dramatically increase your power to take full control over your sleep problems and dramatically enhance your sleep quality. The key to this transition is recognizing that sleep symptoms you previously thought were caused by psychological factors might really be caused or worsened by physical factors. Now you want to pay special attention to symptoms that still bother you and ask yourself:

- Could they be caused by a physiological sleep disorder?
- Is the physical cause greater than a previously perceived mental cause?
- Can I predict whether the symptom will improve with physiological sleep treatment?

COMMENT: Review the following list of symptoms while considering the questions above for any symptom still bothering you. Remember, you just worked diligently on a psychological sleep treatment program, yet many of the following symptoms persist somewhat or more, surely a conundrum to sleep on:

- disturbing dreams or other restless behaviors while sleeping;
- waking up from sleep at night and using the bathroom;
- bed linens in disarray in the morning;
- waking up in the morning with a dry mouth or a headache;
- signs of fatigue or tiredness in your eyes and face;
- sluggish mornings requiring an artificial jump start;
- afternoon dips of energy;
- desiring naps even if you don't nap or can't doze off;
- relying on caffeine to ward off sleepiness, tiredness, or fatigue;
- small improvements in concentration, memory, or attention span;
- no increase in motivation to exercise;
- scant improvement in exercise endurance;
- not losing weight;
- no signs of reductions in your blood pressure.

For two special types of cases, think carefully about the following:

- For known heart patients, do you still suffer poor control of conges- tive heart failure, cardiac arrhythmias, or angina, especially during sleep?
- For known mental health patients who have tried multiple drugs for anxiety, PTSD, or depression, do you still suffer from persisting symptoms of these mental conditions?

All of the above can be and frequently are caused or worsened by undi- agnosed and untreated physiological sleep disorders! In sum, it will greatly speed up your care if you are already contemplating the possibilities link- ing certain of your mental and physical health complaints to physical sleep disorders.

────── PEARL ──────

The Missing Links to Physical Sleep Disorders

Although you and your physician might offer other explanations for these signs and symptoms of poor health, soon you will learn how a single, physical sleep disorder wreaks large-scale havoc on your health. Which reminds me of my favorite Sherlock Holmes quote: "When you have eliminated the impossible, whatever remains, however improbable, must be the truth."

As you read ahead, prepare to meet the improbable!

PART SIX

AWAKEN THE SLUMBERING GIANT

Breathe Your Way to Perfect Sleep Quality

Traveling to a New Dimension

Imagine meeting someone who had never tasted chocolate. Assuming you just savored your last piece, what could you possibly tell him that might convey the taste, texture, flavor, smell, and delicious qualities that encompass a great piece of chocolate?

Your best reply would be: "I can't explain; you just have to taste it."

Which is true of *Sound Sleep*: you just need to taste it.

How much *Sound Sleep* have you tasted in this Sleep Dynamic Therapy (SDT) program? How much have you slowed down your brain waves at bedtime and during the night? Do you have any sense whether you are increasing or consolidating delta (more restorative sleep) or REM (more dream awareness sleep), the two most essential sleep stages? Are you decreasing your amount of stage 1 NREM, the lightest sleep that leads to more awakenings and fragmentation? In short, are you getting the sleep you need?

As you are about to learn, nothing may be more powerful in your efforts to feel the *Day Is Done* experience and to recruit the *Wave of Sleepiness* than to reverse the physiological influences breaking up your sleep, which will then optimize your sleep quality.

This pathway is so important and so critical that all of parts six and seven deal with just three physical sleep disorders, because these are the culprits most likely hidden from your awareness and most likely generating so much sleep fragmentation. You may never attain *Sound Sleep* until you put these sleep disorders to rest.

21

To Breathe, Perchance to Sleep

Take a Breather

Sound sleep is impossible without good breathing . . . while you are sleeping!

You might imagine all sorts of things to persuade yourself that your breathing is normal; but remember, you are asleep when you are asleep. You cannot judge whether your sleep breathing is normal. To demonstrate the importance of a breathing disorder, let's consider two predictions:

1. If you suffer from chronic insomnia or poor sleep quality, you have a 90 percent chance of suffering from a sleep breathing problem.
2. For those with a physiological sleep disorder, more than 50 percent of your sleeplessness is a result of the breathing condition, and don't be surprised if the influence turns out to be greater than that.

Neither you nor your regular doctor would typically suspect this condition or predict its destructive influence on your sleep. Because most troubled sleepers and health-care professionals think of sleeplessness in psychological terms, this new idea feels surprising, confusing, or threatening. I hope you feel a sense of relief and enthusiasm, because diagnosing and treating this problem might resolve your remaining sleep problems.

Say "sleep breathing disorder," and many think of snoring, gasping, choking, and stopping breathing (apnea). These extreme breathing symptoms are the tip of an iceberg, beneath which lie other forms of sleep breathing patterns you'll learn about shortly. What you must know now is that sleep breathing problems destroy slumber in ways more serious and severe than almost any other psychological cause of sleeplessness. If you react skeptically to this new information and believe that breathing could not be your problem, hold that breath—er, thought, feeling, or image—because you just might be headed for a life-changing as well as a life-saving experience.

Connecting the *Zzzots* Again

How important is the knowledge that you might suffer from sleep-disordered breathing (SDB)? Except for very mild to moderate insomnia patients and occasional severe insomniacs, Sleep Dynamic Therapy has never cured nor optimized the sleep of any patient through the exclusive use of psychological treatments, including cognitive-behavioral therapies, imagery skills, and sleep-related emotional processing. Only when SDB also was treated was *Sound Sleep* optimally achieved.

SNOOZE FLASH

Waking Up to Sleep-Disordered Breathing

In more than a decade of clinical experience, working with several thousand insomnia patients as well as those complaining of Poor Sleep Quality, 90 percent never imagined sleep breathing as an influential factor in their complaints. Yet greater than 90 percent were diagnosed with sleep-disordered breathing (SDB), a broad term commonly used in the field of sleep medicine, which serves as an umbrella under which resides different types of conditions.

In many cases, SDB proved the prime cause or a major contributor to their sleeplessness. Unequivocally, SDB was the single most important factor waking them up at night and an aggravating factor in preventing return to sleep. Many of these sleep patients also suffered from mental health problems, which they believed were the only explanations for their sleep disturbances until they learned about SDB. The biggest shock for some of those with psychiatric conditions was that SDB treatment not only decreased insomnia but also improved mental health.

With psychological treatments, patients decreased the time to fall asleep, decreased the number of awakenings, and improved sleep quality, but to teach them consistently:

- how to fall asleep in less than ten minutes;
- how to decrease their awakenings at night to none or maybe one;
- how to roll over and go right back to sleep after any awakening; and
- how to dramatically decrease daytime sleepiness and fatigue and enhance daytime energy,

we needed to treat their SDB. That's how important this information might be for you. Successful treatment of SDB may be the silver bullet many have dreamed about in the hopes of conquering their sleep problems.

The floor is now open for questions:

- Why would a breathing problem cause sleep problems?
- Wouldn't it be obvious if I had a sleep breathing problem?
- How and why would someone develop a sleep breathing problem?
- Does the breathing problem have something to do with stress?
- Why do people who suffer from anxiety, depression, or PTSD also suffer from SDB?
- How much does SDB affect my problems with falling asleep, staying asleep, or waking up unrested?
- If SDB is so common, why hasn't my doctor discussed it with me?
- And last but not least, surely you don't mean I have sleep apnea?

We will answer all these questions.

Gotta Go, Gotta Go

Daytime fatigue, tiredness, and sleepiness remain the three most important symptoms to monitor when measuring the impact of SDB, but we must also look at new symptoms to assess this physiological disorder of respiration, some of which will surprise and amaze you. A common symptom reported by poor sleepers or insomniacs with SDB is waking up at night to use the bathroom. For some, this symptom appears mildly annoying because they easily go back to sleep. For others, using the bathroom wakes them enough to cause difficulty returning to sleep for anywhere from thirty minutes to two hours or longer.

Regardless of how this symptom—called nocturia—affects your sleep, here's something you must know immediately, which you typically do *not* hear from health-care providers: nocturia is not normal. It is a symptom of something, and a tremendous number of problematic sleepers who wake up to urinate at night suffer from SDB, the physiological disorder of respiration, which causes their nocturia.

When this fact is offered to most problematic sleepers, they attempt to explain away their bathroom visits with one of the following:

1. I drink a lot of water at bedtime.
2. I don't get up to pee; I just wake up anyway and choose to pee.
3. It's probably a medicine I'm taking.
4. My doctor says my prostate's enlarged.
5. My doctor says I have a small or a sensitive bladder.
6. My therapist says my anxiety is giving me a nervous bladder.

Many of these factors are relevant. Yet among problematic sleepers, a huge number discover that nocturia decreases or resolves entirely by treating SDB. To let this soak in, let's look at the technical details of sleep-disordered breathing. After this description, you will see the logic and the science as well as the common sense that explains why an SDB patient wakes up at night to urinate more than a normal sleeper. Here's a hint: the kidneys of an SDB patient produce more urine at night than in normal sleepers!

Don't Hold Your Breath

Breathing is the most vital physiological function you must perform to live. The evidence is simple. If you stop breathing for more than a few minutes, not only would you likely die, but if revived with artificial respiration, you might suffer severe and permanent brain damage. Your mind-body is well programmed to recognize the critical function of breathing. Any breathing disruption rapidly triggers your brain to analyze the problem; then, in seconds, your nervous system cues your body to respond to preserve itself.

"Bad breath" drives you to take a "good breath" to restore normal breathing.

Why would this response be so instantaneous and so powerful? Obviously, not breathing could be interpreted by the brain as a life-threatening situation that must be reversed quickly. Consider for a moment your worst fears. Suppose you suffer from a fear of closed spaces (claustrophobia), a fear of heights (acrophobia), a fear of financial ruin, or a fear of losing a loved one. None of these fears can match the physiological intensity of the fear enveloping your mind and body when suddenly choking or suffocating. Not one!

As seconds tick off, only one thought/feeling/image grips you: "I am going to die if I don't start breathing again." Your mind-body responds with every ounce of energy to breathe again. Nothing on Earth generates the magnitude of fear that explodes within while suffocating. This response is healthy, natural, and outstanding evolution, because:

No breath = no life.

The sensors in your mind-body activate any conceivable strategy to respond to breathing distortions, whether awake or asleep. You may respond in as little as a few seconds or less if awake. While asleep, if you experience what the brain perceives as a minisuffocation—a simple restriction in breathing that is not life-threatening—your mind-body still responds quickly. If breathing disruption worsens to no breath at all—apnea—the body wishes to respond faster, but depending on how many years you suffered from sleep apnea, you could stop breathing for thirty to sixty seconds before normal breathing resumes.

First Responses

What exactly is this response to restore normal breathing? What could your mind and body do to make you breathe better while you sleep? Make a guess:

1. The brain sends a nerve impulse to make you breathe better.
2. Your body moves to a different position to breathe better.
3. The mind-body releases something in the blood to improve breathing.

These common answers are all accurate to a degree; however, the question is tricky, because the mind-body can only do so much to resolve breathing problems while you continue sleeping. Above all else, the most complete answer is: brain waves appear to speed up to wake you up, which then enables you to breathe better, because according to human physiology, all people breathe better while awake.

But "if the brain wakes me up, why don't I remember it?" You do sometimes. If you suffer from insomnia or poor sleep quality, you rarely sleep through the night. When you awaken at night, though, you rarely know the cause for the awakening . . . except now you do!

No matter how difficult this idea is to accept, please consider that the most common causes of awakenings are breathing irregularities, which trigger your brain to wake, presumably to take a better breath. You have scant awareness for these wake-ups, because you awaken for as short as 1.5 seconds to up to 60 seconds; then, in most instances, you return to sleep. Do you think you would remember such short arousals or awakenings?

Total Lack of Recall

In research studies testing the capacity to distinguish or remember awakenings from sleep, most people needed to be awake for one to eight minutes after an awakening to recall it. In SDB, the overwhelming majority of wake-ups are less than thirty seconds, and many arousals are only a few seconds. Your mind and memory are not activated long enough to recall this recurring problem.

Brain waves speed up due to disrupted breathing in the ways previously described:

- awakenings (more than 15 seconds);
- arousals (3 to 15 seconds);
- microarousals (1.5 to 3 seconds).

If someone woke you from sleep and invited you to a noon lunch at your favorite restaurant, but you rolled over and went right back to sleep, it's doubtful you'd show up even though you "heard" the invitation. But here's the catch: if after the brief awakening you ruminate about the lunch meeting or something else, which then cascades into racing thoughts, your mind grows increasingly more awake. Soon the experience becomes a memorable awakening, if not the start of insomnia, and then you would recall the lunch date.

Let Me Count the Ways

This brings us to a big question.

"How many times could I be suffering from these arousals or awakenings from SDB . . . and not know it?" Before you guess, please grasp that you only remember a few awakenings during the night—the ones where you ruminated about something after you woke yourself.

Now consider these facts:

- Most people while sleeping take about ten to eighteen breaths each minute.
- If we use an average of 12 breaths a minute for 60 minutes, we calculate 720 breaths per hour.
- If you sleep 6 hours a night, we calculate as many as 4,320 breaths during a single night's sleep.
- Last fact: if your breathing becomes disrupted, even slightly, the brain can respond after as few as two or three "bad breaths" to fix the problem.

Now do the math: how many times might you arouse or awaken during the night? For most poor sleepers with SDB, you arouse or awaken hundreds of times, usually between 200 and 500 per night. The problem, though, is much worse than this astonishing number of wake-ups. The fragmenting effect on your sleep kicks you out of or prevents you from entering deeper stages of sleep such as delta or REM, which causes you to spend too much time in stage 1 NREM. With SDB triggering the brain to speed up, you receive less sleep overall, more lighter stages of sleep, and ultimately worse sleep quality.

Making matters still worse, sleep fragmentation itself interferes with breathing. The arousal activity designed to help you breathe better triggers a cycle of lighter sleep, after which your breathing destabilizes again. That is, in stage 1 NREM, you are more prone to SDB events. Please keep this fact in mind if you suffer from mental health problems, because it's distinctly possible that your emotional distress lightens your sleep and thus worsens your breathing.

In Comes the Good Air

Do you see how much closer we are to a complete explanation of *Poor Sleep Quality*? SDB is the absolute best example of how you might perceive sleeping eight hours, when in fact disrupted breathing sped up your brain, leaving you with a total sleep time of only four to six hours.

SDB is the leading cause of poor sleep quality because it literally robs you of slumber and degrades the sleep left behind in its wake. Yet you have no memory of the thievery unfolding in your bedroom, night after night, and you certainly don't know where or how to place the blame for these crimes against your sleep.

If you were arousing or awakening all night long and not entering deeper stages of sleep, it ought to be crystal clear that your sleep no longer restores you each night, which explains perfectly your feelings of sleepiness, tiredness, and fatigue the next day. SDB may be the ultimate monster that destroys your sleep quality! But this monster is incredibly deceptive, because SDB neither slaps you on the side of the head in the morning nor reveals itself when you awaken unrefreshed. It is a silent, disabling, and sometimes deadly monster.

To demonstrate the far-reaching grip that SDB has over mind and body, a grip so tight it affects your mental and physical health, let's clarify how it causes nocturia.

Listen to Your Kidneys

Your cardiovascular system contains a volume of fluid within the heart and its connecting blood vessels, also called the circulatory system. The kidneys draw fluid out of this system to regulate the fluid level. If the volume is too high (fluid overload), blood pressure could go too high. If the volume is too low (dehydration), blood pressure could drop. The kidneys respond to either situation by pulling more or less fluid from the system, which means producing more or less urine—urine output—to maintain correct circulatory volume and proper blood pressure.

During sleep, a normal sleeper sleeps through the night without taking in any fluid. What should the kidneys do? If no fluid comes in, the kidneys generate less urine to maintain proper hydration in the bloodstream. Thus, urine output decreases during sleep, so unless another problem arises, normal sleepers don't use the bathroom at night.

Enter SDB.

The obstruction or resistance to breathing in your upper airway causes your chest to work much harder than during normal breathing. During this struggle for breath, the body exerts more effort to pull air into the lungs, and this causes a large change in pressure inside the chest cavity. This change in pressure has an unexpected side effect that forces more blood to flow toward the heart. The increased blood flow enters the right atrium of the heart, stretching the muscles in this chamber. Can you guess how these heart muscle cells interpret stretching?

Go to the head of the class if you said, "the heart detects this change as a sign of fluid overload." The right atrium perceives a direct threat to the body, and it must do something quickly to counteract this signal of a fluid-overload state. Any guess what?

Two gold stars if you said, "it must send a signal to the kidneys to make more urine to relieve the fluid overload." In fact, the right atrial heart muscles release a hormone known as atrial natriuretic peptide (ANP) into the bloodstream, which is a diuretic—something that makes the kidneys produce more urine. In controlled research studies, patients with SDB produced more ANP and more urine than normal sleepers did.

For those whose bladders might be small or sensitive or nervous, can you see how it takes only a small increase in urine output to trigger the need to pee?

As intriguing as the explanation for nocturia sounds, the more amazing fact is that successfully treated SDB rapidly and dramatically reduces ANP and urine output on the first night of treatment. SDB patients who respond to treatment report fewer or no trips to the bathroom at night. Can you imagine that—not going to the bathroom once, just by treating SDB?

Surely these ideas are something to sleep on . . . all through the night!

SLEEP ON IT
Take a Deep Breath

QUESTION: After hearing about SDB, most problematic sleepers wish to know whether this physical condition afflicts them. But ambivalent feelings also arise, because few can imagine how to treat it. If someone you know uses a breathing mask therapy, you might be anxious that a mask is the only option . . . but let's not jump ahead. Before clarifying treatment steps in the upcoming Sleep on It sections, we must confirm whether and how much SDB affects your sleep. So: What are your chances of suffering from SDB?

COMMENT: Poor sleepers respond with many answers. For some, it's a revelation. All their speculations about sleep problems fit into a clearer framework, because they always knew something physical damaged their sleep. Learning about SDB is a breath of fresh air. Others nervously accept SDB, but the anxiety about it prevents them from seeing how a very treatable condition causes much of their broken sleep.

Many mental health patients with SDB are elated, because for years they knew sleep problems were not strictly mental, but their doctors or therapists never guided them toward physical causes. However, some mental health patients feel overwhelmed by something else being wrong with their health. SDB feels like an added weight instead of a burden lifted; their image focuses on something that's more trouble than it's worth.

Finally, some individuals remain in denial, insisting they do not have SDB. These patients have heard—for too many years—that the only explanations for sleep problems are stress, mental health symptoms, and chemical imbalances. Having heard this view for five, ten, or twenty years, their senses are jarred when asked to consider a physical cause that might be as or more important than psychiatric or psychological ones.

To expedite care for individuals with such varied responses, we find it most helpful to offer preliminary and relatively easy treatments to those with suspected SDB. Hopefully, immediate relief follows from the instructions ahead. Or you may learn new insights to motivate you toward other treatments. If you recognize SDB in yourself and want to pursue advanced treatment now, do not hesitate to schedule an appointment at your local sleep center or sleep lab, because it might take weeks or months to see a sleep specialist.

———— PEARL ————
The Knock-Your-Socks-off Rapid SDB Diagnostic Tool

Nailing down the SDB diagnosis is our first step. Some make the diagnosis quickly if they become aware of obvious sleep breathing symptoms, such as snoring, gasping, or choking. However, many people with insomnia or poor sleep quality have limited awareness of breathing symptoms.

Here's an indirect and simpler way to spot the likelihood of this disorder. Tonight, place a pair of socks at the end of your bed, about a foot or two from the edge. When you awaken in the morning, determine the whereabouts of the socks. Repeat this instruction for a few nights to see whether a pattern emerges. Many poor sleepers toss and turn at night and find their sheets and blankets in disarray in the morning, which is not a sign of normal sleep. You may wake up in an unusual spot on the bed or notice your body in a twisted position. A pair of socks at the end of your bed should still be there in the morning. If the socks were pushed off the bed, then your tossing and turning or the movements of your legs at night have gone far beyond normal sleep. You likely suffer from one of two conditions.

SDB is the most common cause for tossing and turning, because you are attempting to reposition yourself to breathe better. But no perfect position solves your breathing problem, so you keep moving. The second possibility is a sleep movement condition in which your legs twitch, jerk, or move too much while you sleep.

Regardless of the cause, this excessive movement is not normal and rarely is caused by mental factors. Instead, physical factors are the leading causes of restless sleep.

If you use medication to sleep, you might toss and turn less, but few of these medicines improve breathing or leg movements. Some sedatives may worsen breathing, and some antidepressants worsen leg movements. Moreover, using these medications might inadvertently lead you astray in your efforts to diagnose this part of your sleep problem.

Again, we are faced with the dilemma that you cannot watch yourself move during sleep, and your instincts tend to normalize your tossing-and-turning behavior. This brings us to the single most commonly normalized abnormal sleep behavior: snoring.

22

The Anti-Sandman:
The Sequel

Snoring Is Boring

From the sleep medicine perspective, snoring is a tedious and surprisingly complex issue upon which most time spent is largely wasted. We ask patients few questions about snoring, because it is a relatively worthless symptom to analyze for a sleep-disordered breathing (SDB) diagnosis.

More pertinent, snoring issues erect barriers to the treatment of sleep problems because:

- few people can detect their own snoring;
- most honestly do not know if they snore;
- many lie or minimize what they know about their snoring;
- snoring is embarrassing, so people don't discuss it;
- snoring clearly injures the sleep of others in your bedroom;
- talking about snoring triggers emotions of anger, guilt, or shame;
- snoring is often absent when SDB is diagnosed in a sleep lab;
- there is no clear scientific definition or measurement of snoring;
- you don't have to snore to suffer from SDB.

This last barrier is spread through perniciously inadequate media coverage on television, radio, in print, or in Internet formats, which offer useless and sometimes dangerous information about your health. Let me underscore dangerous, because these superficial media pieces lead people away from proper sleep evaluations by feeding the lie that snoring must be present to suffer from SDB. Even children with SDB don't necessarily snore. Adding to this problem, poor sleepers who request help from primary-care physicians are often advised, "without snoring, there can be no SDB."

In sleep medicine, we discuss snoring so you don't become confused about the meaning or significance of snoring. For example, snoring is easily defined as vibrations of soft palate tissue during respiration, but SDB patients can make all types of noises with their breathing while asleep. Noises include snores, snorts, gasps, chokes, nasal whistles, heavy breathing, and rapid breathing, and these sounds come in all colors and flavors. You could measure the intensity, duration, pitch, frequency, consistency, and even the likely origin of the noise, but none of this information guarantees the presence or absence of SDB. Granted, the noisier you breathe, your chances skyrocket for severe SDB. But SDB patients can also make no special noises.

Snoring is also unreliable because many loud snorers, particularly premenopausal women, do not show much apnea, but instead show subtle forms of SDB disturbances. And snoring is frequently absent in the sleep lab when patients are tested, yet SDB is still diagnosed in mild, moderate, or severe forms.

Turning Red . . .

Embarrassment is arguably the biggest snoring issue. Just watch someone's face when you ask "Do you snore?" Talk about mind-body language. Few people respond with candid or comfortable answers. Most exhibit an immediate reaction of discomfort, including a nervous laugh, a twitchy face, aversion of the eyes, a perplexed look, or a sudden impulse to provide rambling answers like "Well, you know, I don't think so, but my wife says differently, and there was that time at the campground when the kids wanted to bury me alive, but no, I really don't think I snore very much . . . well, maybe a little, but not at all like my family imagines . . . I guess."

Parts four and five taught you to develop emotional processing skills while learning to appreciate how emotions always win! Snoring issues are perfect examples of how troubled sleepers say or act in a useless way when driven by their emotions. Many sleep patients hide from any discussion of snoring because they fear embarrassment, shame, or guilt. Why would they feel this way? Because one person's snoring damages or interferes with another person's sleep. The injured sleeper is in the same bed or bedroom, but the snorer has no awareness of this unintentional harm to the other sleeper. Once the topic is broached, the snorer feels embarrassed or guilty about having done something without any awareness of doing it.

If snoring persists for years, the relationship at night can turn sour, and the snorer feels ashamed of this behavior. Many cannot imagine snoring being such a serious matter producing such intense feelings. But snoring and sleep breathing problems are serious business, which, based on scientific studies, cause sufficient marital disharmony to lead people toward estrangement, separation, or divorce.

Some SDB patients must overcome embarrassment about snoring or other noisy or troublesome breathing behaviors before they can move forward with treatment. Using emotional processing skills is the fastest way to do so. Healthy emotional processors welcome the chance to sleep better and recognize that treating the condition eliminates the source of embarrassment.

. . . Then Yellow

Many undiagnosed SDB patients or those who snore suffer other medical conditions that previously threatened their lives. A cardiac patient recovering from a heart attack or a trauma survivor recovering from an assault are not eager to discuss snoring or the possibility of a new sleep diagnosis. Their nerves may have been unsettled for months or years, leaving them on guard about undesirable health news. Fear is the primary feeling that cardiac or trauma patients would do well to identify and work through, but instead many find themselves caught up in anxiety. Ironically, even the smallest of breathing discomfort, awake or asleep, triggers more anxiety in these patients.

A sizable minority of sleep patients cannot tap into any feelings about snoring or SDB; they flat-out reject the information and have no intention of evaluating or treating it. Make no mistake about it: the inability to connect with pertinent feelings triggered by the discovery of a snoring problem or an SDB diagnosis prevents many troubled sleepers from attaining *Sound Sleep*.

Indeed, many people lie about snoring. Many more honestly do not know whether they snore. Snoring and breathing symptoms raise complex issues, which provide few answers and more hassle when diagnosing and treating SDB. Beware of putting too much focus on breathing symptoms, because you have limited capacity to monitor these signs. Once you visit a sleep center, your breathing symptoms can be objectively measured in a sleep lab.

> **SNOOZE FLASH**
> ## Never Underestimate the Meaning of Snoring
> Despite the conventional wisdom, snoring is a nearly universal sign of airway obstruction. With the latest respiratory technology, it is now apparent that most snoring is a sign of frequent mini-suffocations that result in numerous microarousals, arousals, or even awakenings. If you snore, assume you have some SDB, but currently you will not find many physicians who agree with these facts.

Don't Wait to Lose Weight

Finally, obesity is a critical factor most poor sleepers and health-care providers link to snoring and SDB. Yet, in our field, we repeatedly hear stories from nonobese or nonoverweight SDB patients (of whom there are tens of millions) whose primary-care physicians advised against a sleep center visit, declaring it a waste of time. These patients or physicians were misinformed, because obesity rarely causes SDB; rather, it makes SDB worse. Even when SDB patients lose enough pounds to reach normal weight, SDB severity may decrease, but rarely is it cured.

Some medical professionals encourage patients to lose weight instead of seeking help at sleep centers. This view is misguided because many other factors create risks for SDB, the two most important of which are:

- genetic (whether or not your blood relatives suffer from SDB);
- the anatomy of your airway, which is based on genetics; development in childhood; development in adolescence; nutrition; breast-feeding; current dentition; current weight; history of lost or extracted teeth; orthodontic history; physical obstructions such as a deviated septum, sinus blockage, or polyps; traumatic injuries to head, face, or neck; or past nasal or oral surgeries.

The size and shape of your head and of various internal airway structures are the most important physical factors determining SDB. Many obese patients show crowded tissues inside the airway, but few primary-care physicians pay attention to precise airway structures. Weight loss is useful for some SDB patients, but we recommend simultaneous treatment of the sleep breathing condition.

SLEEP ON IT
No Tongue Blades Needed

QUESTIONS: Many SDB patients develop a sense about their airway long before finding out they have SDB, because they notice:

- difficulty swallowing pills;
- accidentally biting the sides of their tongue or their cheeks;
- occasionally choking on food;
- a clear feeling that it's difficult to breathe while awake.

Have you had these experiences? Do you believe your airway might be crowded? Have you experienced any of the items below?

- Did you have several teeth extracted when you were younger, because your dental arches were said to be crowded?
- Did you wear orthodontic headgear or strap-on rubber bands to hold back the growth of the maxilla (upper jaw) so the mandible (lower jaw) would catch up to correct an overbite?
- Did you have your tonsils removed too late to affect growth of the airway (that is, after age two)?
- Did you break your nose and never have it evaluated?

COMMENT: Airway crowding involves two primary components. First, facial structure comes from your mother or your father's side of the family. If one parent has a vertically shaped or narrow head, as opposed to a square or round shape, and you inherited a narrow face, your airway is more likely to be crowded. A narrow head yields a longish-looking face and may include a small chin. This combination signals less space in the area of the lower jaw and usually results in airway crowding or a smaller airway.

The second component involves the inner structure of your airway. Nasal airflow is critical to good breathing. A deviated septum reduces airflow to the back of the throat. If your hard palate (the roof of your mouth) is narrow and pushes up into the nasal cavity, less space is available for air to pass through the nose. Last, the back of the tongue may be thick and ride high toward the back of the throat, covering up the airway. This degree of crowding is seen with classic sleep apnea. However, something that looks crowded does not necessarily mean that it acts in a crowded way. Your airway structures are dynamic, so what you see is not necessarily what you get.

—————— PEARL ——————
The Nasal-Oral Airway Exam Made Easy

A few minutes spent looking at your face, nose, and airway may yield important clues about your breathing. The pictures on pages 220 and 221 help to identify important oral structures.

Stand in front of a mirror with good lighting. Use a flashlight, too. Begin by gently pinching your nostrils, then let one side open and breathe naturally, without forcing or laboring air through that nostril. Then close off that nostril and open the other one. Go back and forth until you determine that the volume and relative force of breathing through each nostril is about equal or not. Next, put your index and middle finger on the tip of your nose and gently push it upward. Using the flashlight, see if the space inside one nostril looks smaller or larger than the other and whether the midline cartilage (the septum) is tilted or bulging to one side. Notice whether you seem congested in your nasal breathing. Many people suffer low-grade stuffiness due to allergies or dryness, which may affect breathing more than they suspect.

Now peer inside your open mouth but don't say "Ahhh!" Look around at all the structures, top and bottom. Open your mouth and stick out your tongue, but again don't say "Ahhh!" Usually you see a portion of the airway opening. If you cannot see any opening, the two most likely factors are related to your soft palate or uvula (the dangly tissue at the end of the soft palate) or the base (back) of your tongue. Excessive soft palate tissue, hanging down into the back of your throat, covers up the top of the airway opening; and in a few cases, the soft palate is so floppy it covers most of the airway. Some surgeons perform a procedure to remove this tissue (uvulo-palato-pharyngoplasty, UPPP), which I advise against as a first-line treatment. UPPP not only has a mediocre success rate, but also emerging evidence suggests that UPPP worsens some SDB cases or makes it difficult to use other treatment options. Rarely is it a curative procedure for SDB, even if it stops the snoring.

When examining the soft palate, take note of the uvula; if elongated, thickened, or red, it indicates you snore or your breathing encounters lots of friction along these passages, which

Chart 3. Oral Airway Structures

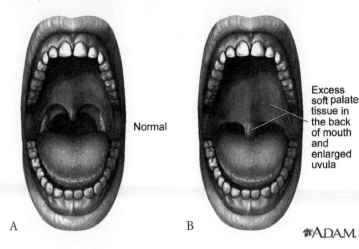

Normal

Excess
soft palate
tissue in
the back
of mouth
and
enlarged
uvula

A   B   ✿A.D.A.M.

Picture A. Normal Airway
The four main structures are the tongue, soft palate, uvula (dangly tissue drooping from the middle of the soft palate), and tonsils on each side of the airway. Note how easily you see the airway. The back or base of the tongue does not ride up high to cover the airway. The soft palate or uvula does not extend downward to cover it. The tonsils do not push in toward the middle to cover it.

Picture B. Excessive Soft Palate Tissue
The uvula is swollen and the soft palate is enlarged, both now hanging so far into the back of the throat, they reduce the size of the airway by more than half. Unfortunately, surgery on the soft palate and uvula often produces mixed or poor results in SDB patients, sometimes worsening SDB severity and sometimes making it very difficult for the patient to ever successfully use the breathing mask treatment (PAP therapy).

irritates and swells the tissues. Snoring vibration produces similar damage.

In some, the base of the tongue rides high in the back of the throat and covers up the bottom of the airway opening or higher up. When the whole opening is covered by either or both the tongue or soft palate, the airway is deemed very crowded and at potentially high risk for SDB, particularly apnea. However, this exam is not always reliable, because many patients with severe crowding show no apnea in the sleep lab. Instead, subtle forms of breathing disturbance may be seen that still require aggressive treatment.

Chart 3. Oral Airway Structures (continued)

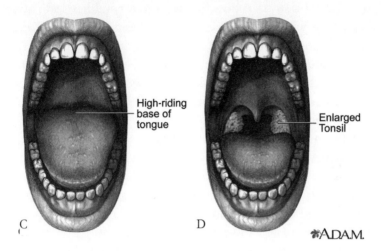

Picture C. High-Riding Tongue Base
The tongue is now thickened at the back of the throat or simply rides up too high, covering up most of the airway. You can barely see the top of the airway: two very small openings situated on either side of where the tongue base covers the uvula. This degree of tongue crowding often predicts severe SDB.

Picture D. Enlarged Tonsils
The tonsils are very large and crowd toward the middle of the airway. In some cases, especially in kids, the tonsils are so large, they "kiss" in the middle. Surgical removal of tonsils in children is a reliable technique to reduce SDB severity. In adults with enlarged tonsils, SDB severity also decreases in most cases following surgery, but you must be forewarned about the post-operative period, during which you may suffer severe pain.

The more you learn about SDB, the more you will find yourself wanting to test your breathing or swallowing. If such steps make you nervous, don't bother, but if you are curious about your breathing, make mental notes on your observations. Spend most of your initial efforts examining your nasal breathing, because if you find problems there, you can try some very simple treatment steps.

On the other hand, some people feel nervous or fearful about the exam and develop anxiety about whether SDB patients can choke to death in their sleep. All the scientific evidence suggests that choking to death during sleep is rare, because our evolution has programmed us to have a strong drive to restart breathing if it stops. A possible scenario for sudden death arises in patients with serious heart disease. When their oxygen levels drop during SDB episodes, a life-threatening cardiac rhythm disturbance can be triggered. If you believe you suffer from a severe form of SDB as well as from serious heart or lung problems, then inform your doctor to arrange for rapid evaluation at a sleep center.

The overwhelming majority of SDB patients do not require emergency attention, and this point is intended to ease anxieties as you learn more about SDB and look more closely at your airway. Some with SDB and severe sleepiness are at high risk for car crashes, and these individuals are advised to stop driving until their SDB is treated, but again, the vast majority of SDB patients do not appear to require urgent treatment. Then again, the wait at many sleep centers is measured in months, so it never hurts to get on the waiting list.

23

Waking Up to Better Breathing

Making the Diagnosis

The only reliable way to diagnose sleep-disordered breathing (SDB) is in the sleep lab. You could also confirm crowded features in your airway and link them to obvious disruption in breathing. Although these steps are reliable, they may be inconvenient right now. Your next diagnostic option would link sleep symptoms directly to a sleep fragmentation problem such as SDB or leg movements. Most have already made this sleep fragmentation connection because they acknowledge symptoms of poor sleep quality, unrefreshing sleep, daytime sleepiness or tiredness, and a desire to nap during the day. Perhaps you are still not persuaded that these symptoms mark the presence of SDB.

We help patients overcome this skepticism by offering two other ways for making a rapid presumptive SDB diagnosis. The word "presumptive" means we can't be 100 percent certain until the sleep test is performed, but we can predict with near-certainty.

Count Your Symptoms

At our sleep centers, we find that most patients will report some of the sleep quality problems mentioned above, particularly the presence of daytime fatigue or sleepiness, but to confirm an SDB diagnosis, we find these six symptoms the most reliable:

1. waking up from sleep at any time with a dry mouth;
2. nocturia;
3. waking up in the morning with a headache;
4. impaired concentration;
5. impaired memory;
6. difficulty paying attention.

Once a patient reports four of these symptoms, we find an extraordinarily high rate of SDB. Yet, as I'm sure you noticed, none of these symptoms looks much like a specific sleep complaint. Instead, these problems are known as "end organ" symptoms—that is, they reflect how SDB targets and damages various organ systems in the body.

What's fascinating about these symptoms is that many other medical diseases might cause them. In actuality, there are not that many unique conditions that cause all six. For example, most physicians might immediately think of diabetes, but this deadly disease does not typically cause morning headaches; and the cognitive impairment in diabetes is variable, whereas virtually all SDB patients demonstrate fairly obvious mild to severe cognitive impairment due to sleep fragmentation. And this impair-

---

SNOOZE FLASH

SDB Diagnoses Made without Breathing Symptoms

Our research team published a paper in the *Journal of Nervous and Mental Disease* in 2006 that highlights the importance of end-organ symptoms in SDB. The study compared typical sleep apnea patients (group 1) with trauma survivors who suffered SDB (group 2). Most apnea patients knew they snored and reported daytime sleepiness. Nearly all trauma survivors emphasized nighttime insomnia complaints, and only 25 percent thought they snored. Yet all 178 patients (89 in each group) suffered SDB, diagnosed with advanced respiratory technology, yet both groups looked quite different. Virtually any physician would have suspected sleep apnea in the first group, whereas the second group mirrored psychiatric patients suffering insomnia. But when end-organ symptoms were assessed, there were no differences between the groups. Both reported high rates of cognitive impairment, nocturia, and morning headache or dry mouth. These similarities show the value of end-organ symptoms among those without breathing complaints.

ment is much worse if the SDB is compromising blood oxygenation as well.

Another interesting example is depression in which patients might report all six symptoms, particularly cognitive impairment. However, dry mouth, headache, and nocturia could easily be related to antidepressant medication side effects—not the depression—so you must know whether you suffered these symptoms before taking such medication.

Let's not forget the most heralded explanation: getting older! Surely, aging is the cause of all these symptoms; there's no need to look further. Except, when you treat SDB, all six symptoms often improve far beyond any aging treatment ever discovered, invented, or promoted.

End-Organ Symptom Facts

Of these six symptoms, you know how SDB causes nocturia and how sleep fragmentation causes cognitive impairment. Regarding the latter, let me reiterate that the attack on memory, concentration, and attention compromises your capacity to see how SDB cripples your mind. Once again, the monster robs you of the very senses you need to uncover its assault on your sleep.

Now let's talk about waking up with a headache or dry mouth. When a poor sleeper cannot breathe well through the nose, a reflex causes the mouth to open to try to breathe in a greater volume of air through the oral airway. Mouth breathing is a clear sign of airway obstruction, usually in the nose, which leads to dryness in the lips, mouth, tongue, or throat upon awakening.

Morning headaches may be caused by altered blood flow in the brain triggered by fluctuating oxygenation or carbon dioxide levels due to SDB, or possibly frequent repositioning of head and neck to breathe better. Of the six symptoms listed, morning headache is the least common. When you suffer four of six symptoms, they are reliable indicators of a clinically meaningful sleep breathing disorder.

Do-It-Yourself Sleep Diagnosis

The second system to confirm a likely SDB diagnosis would be to treat it and see whether symptoms improve. A magic sleep wand would come in handy here, because the impact of a single night of fully treated SDB confirms the diagnosis to nearly any troubled sleeper the very next day.

There are four major approaches to SDB treatment that progress toward greater intensity, cost, and effort. They also progress toward greater levels of effectiveness and symptom improvement. Some conservative treatments may make a difference, which confirms that you must be suffering from SDB. These are the four options:

1. changing the position of your body while you sleep;
2. aggressive nasal airway therapies;
3. technologically advanced breathing devices;
4. surgery.

Now we'll focus on the first two, which are easy, inexpensive steps.

Placebos

When you use conservative treatments, your results can be driven by a desire to see good results. Placebo is a valid concept, but in my opinion it is often misunderstood and misapplied. If you tried a simple technique for your presumptive SDB, how would you know whether it was a placebo effect if you felt less sleepy the next few days? The answer can almost always be found by asking "How long does the improvement last?"

Placebos rarely last a long time. If you used conservative SDB treatment and noticed that your symptoms were still improving several weeks later, it would be unusual for a placebo to last that long. Once you go beyond one month and improvement is sustained, it would be unlikely for the placebo response to explain these improvements, unless you were involved in a research program that used a technique called "deception" to reinforce the potency of the placebo.

A great deal of recent research shows what most physicians, researchers, and patients have known for a long time: placebo responses on average are not large. Indeed, they are often quite small. None of this information means that placebos should be discredited, and you must be mindful of placebo effects when using conservative treatments. The three most important considerations to bear in mind are:

- Use a technique for at least one month or longer.
- Establish a systematic way to monitor changes during treatment.
- Expect changes to occur in multiple symptoms, not just in one area.

Self-Monitoring

The Sleep-Disordered Breathing-28 questionnaire that follows integrates material from the Sleep Misery Index (page 25) and the Physical Sleep

Sleep-Disordered Breathing-28 Questionnaire

Please answer the following questions, which include critical signs and symptoms linked to sleep-disordered breathing:

	Frequency (How often do you have/feel ...)			
	Never	Sometimes	Often	Always
1. Unrefreshing sleep	☐	☐	☐	☐
2. Restlessness at night	☐	☐	☐	☐
3. Slowed down	☐	☐	☐	☐
4. Acid reflux during the night	☐	☐	☐	☐
5. Low energy during the day	☐	☐	☐	☐
6. Sleepiness during the day	☐	☐	☐	☐
7. Awakenings during the night	☐	☐	☐	☐
8. Too worried about things	☐	☐	☐	☐
9. Anxiety during the day	☐	☐	☐	☐
10. Irritability during the day	☐	☐	☐	☐
11. Decreased activity level	☐	☐	☐	☐
12. Difficulty falling asleep	☐	☐	☐	☐
13. Problems controlling high blood pressure	☐	☐	☐	☐
14. Daytime fatigue or tiredness	☐	☐	☐	☐
15. Difficulty staying asleep	☐	☐	☐	☐
16. Everything is an effort	☐	☐	☐	☐
17. Decreased libido	☐	☐	☐	☐
18. Depression during the day	☐	☐	☐	☐
19. Decreased interest in things	☐	☐	☐	☐
20. Waking up too early	☐	☐	☐	☐
21. Racing thoughts at night	☐	☐	☐	☐
22. Choking or gasping for breath while asleep	☐	☐	☐	☐
23. Difficulty paying attention	☐	☐	☐	☐
24. Difficulty concentrating	☐	☐	☐	☐
25. Memory problems	☐	☐	☐	☐
26. Morning dry mouth	☐	☐	☐	☐
27. Morning headaches	☐	☐	☐	☐
28. Bathroom visits at night	☐	☐	☐	☐

Disturbance Keys (page 200). Because all symptoms listed can be caused by SDB, you can accurately monitor how well treatment is working. You want to see changes in several symptoms to confirm the validity of the changes. The SDB-28 is an outstanding way to monitor progress, and you should use it regularly with the aid of your SOLO skill:

- after trying out any new treatment step for SDB;
- at regular three-month intervals to clarify your progress;
- at least once per year to gain a clear picture for annual checkups.

SLEEP ON IT
Breathe Your Way to Better Sleep

QUESTION: What exactly are we treating when we treat SDB?

COMMENT: No explanation in the scientific literature adequately or completely details all the mechanisms through which a person develops and suffers from SDB. Nonetheless, three active elements can be described:

1. The tongue falls into the back of the throat, blocking the airway during sleep.
2. The anatomy of the oral cavity and throat is crowded, causing resistance when you breathe during sleep.
3. The anatomy of the nasal cavity is crowded, causing resistance when you breathe during sleep.

To take advantage of these facts, we can work in areas to reposition the body during sleep or improve nasal/oral breathing.

Sleep position is important because breathing in adolescents and adults frequently worsens while sleeping on the back. Gravity makes the position worse, presumably by causing the tongue to fall to the back of the throat, inducing obstruction or increasing airway resistance. Research on sleep positions supports sleeping on your side or stomach. Some people may currently avoid sleeping on their back, which clues you in to the diagnosis. When sleep patients swear they cannot sleep on their back, SDB is one likely explanation. The individual has learned a healthy adaptation by sleeping on the stomach or the side, but the larger question is how consistently the individual can maintain these positions throughout the night.

——— PEARL ———
Back "Off" and Decrease SDB Severity

If you sleep on your back, it might be difficult to break the habit, because you must accommodate a change. One motivator for this change is to first experience improved breathing while awake. Just lying down, check out different positions to see which yields easiest breathing. Noticing improvement on your side or stomach raises your confidence to attempt not sleeping on your back. If you want to go low high-tech, the Internet provides a wealth of products to wear that promote *not* sleeping on your back, including tennis balls sewn into a T-shirt, which causes you to roll off your back.

Many people report experiencing a positive elbow sign, usually to the ribs, kidneys, or shoulder from a loving spouse, who is redirecting you to move off your back to stop snoring. However, this sign indicates you have been rolling back onto your back. If you are still unable to completely avoid supine sleep (on the back), you cannot give yourself a good test of this step.

Others want to sleep on their back to decrease joint or back pain. If you find yourself committed to back-sleeping, then shop for special pillows to reposition the neck to improve airflow. Whether these devices work well is debatable. But with a careful search, many people find a device that helps or comforts them, so please consider these options if you must sleep supine.

Last, don't underestimate your own ingenuity in finding solutions because you might create something to avoid sleeping on your back or to reposition your neck. Many people report placing tennis balls in a bra and wearing it front to back.

On the other hand, moving off your back rarely cures SDB, as some patients have as much sleep disruption while sleeping on their sides, and they will need to move on to the next treatment step.

One final note of caution regarding infants. Recent research shows that they should avoid sleeping on their stomachs and should instead attempt to sleep on their backs. This reduces the risk of Sudden Infant Death Syndrom (SIDS). Therefore, avoiding the supine position is not advisable for infants.

24

The Nose Knows

Scoping Things Out

If an ear, nose, and throat (ENT) physician placed a fiberoptic scope through your nose to see the lining of the nasal passages as well as farther along into the nasopharynx—the back of the nasal passages connected to the throat, just behind the soft palate—this exam frequently reveals dried-up mucus stuck to the passages, congestion, or snot.

When the ENT doctor irrigates these regions and sucks out the debris, not only is it a disgusting thing to see and feel, but also it is remarkable how much more clearly you breathe afterward. Most people have more congested debris in their nose and the back of their throat than they realize, even when they know they suffer from allergies and congestion. Few people attend to their nasal breathing aggressively to maximize airflow through the nose. As humans tend to normalize behaviors, they suffer from chronic nasal stuffiness or congestion for years and assume these symptoms don't need evaluation or treatment. If stuffiness worsens, a threshold is passed, which leads to a drugstore to find an over-the-counter remedy. If it worsens further, a large proportion of individuals seek medical advice, which results in prescription medications and prescription nasal sprays.

To treat sleep-disordered breathing and clarify a diagnosis, nasal breathing must be maximized. Just the slightest untreated allergies, congestion, or stuffiness compromises your efforts to treat SDB. Often, aggressive treatment optimizing nasal breathing produces dramatic improvements in sleep symptoms by literally reducing the severity of SDB.

When you consider the following steps, pay close attention to whether you have been prone to normalizing your nasal breathing.

The Power of Salt Water

Before starting, obtain a squeeze bottle of nasal saline spray from your pharmacy. Or obtain a suction bulb and make a solution of one-half cup of warm water and one-half teaspoon of salt (preferably without additives). Carry out these next steps for a few uninterrupted minutes near bedtime.

Station yourself in a bathroom with a sink and a shower. First, sit quietly and listen to and feel your nasal breathing. Notice if you hear a nasal whistle or other sign of congestion. If you suffer from obvious allergies, you will easily see and feel the congestion.

Now use the nasal saline spray while bending over the bathroom sink, and spend a few minutes cleaning out your nose. This step can be combined with a hot shower, during which, if you can safely manage it, sit or stand out of the shower spray and turn the temperature hot enough to generate steam. Please don't burn yourself!

In the shower, initiate or repeat your use of the nasal saline spray to thoroughly clean out your nostrils again, which requires blowing or picking your nose. Most people discover mucus or other debris coming out of the nostrils. Once out of the shower and dried off, sit quietly again and listen and feel your nasal breathing. Most people notice a change for the better, with greater ease of breathing. Check this procedure out for a couple of days before moving on to the next step, and consider washing out your nose at least twice a day, first thing in the morning and within thirty minutes of going to sleep.

Ramping Up Your Nasal Breathing

The exact percentage of SDB patients with allergies is unknown but is suspected to be 70 percent to 80 percent; a sizable but smaller percentage suffer from sinus conditions. One theory to explain this preponderance of allergy and sinus problems is that SDB irritates and inflames tissues in the nasal and oral airways. This inflammation occurs through air turbulence or vibrations (snoring) that arise during problematic sleep breathing. Many SDB patients must aggressively use nasal cleansing and antiallergy treatments weeks before using advanced breathing treatments. In fact, among those using the breathing mask treatment CPAP—continuous positive airway pressure that pushes air into the airway to prevent collapse— the added air may aggravate allergies or sinus conditions, especially among those with a less common condition known as nonallergic or vasomotor rhinitis. In this condition, various stimuli such as wind, temperature, weather changes, environmental irritants, or even saline rinses can stuff up the nose.

Most patients respond to Nasalcrom, an over-the-counter spray for the treatment of certain allergies. Many SDB patients also need prescription treatments, including antihistamine medicines or nasal steroid sprays. Ramping up your treatment of nasal congestion, allergies, and stuffiness through every means possible is an absolute must for SDB patients. One caution: don't use sprays advertising instant relief. Such sprays cause side effects when used on a daily basis, including worse congestion when you stop using them.

Putting together a plan for aggressive nasal hygiene takes patience. At the extreme are individuals with severe sinus and allergy problems or vasomotor rhinitis markedly aggravated by SDB. These patients benefit from consultation with an allergist or an ENT physician. They should also consider at-home irrigation tools to regularly rinse out nasal passages. Keeping these areas cleaned out not only prevents sinus problems, but also this cleansing aids any current treatment of an acute allergy or sinus condition. Vasomotor rhinitis patients must be careful not to aggravate their nasal congestion with these tools and should work closely with an allergist.

Many individuals with less severe conditions benefit from nasal saline washes, Nasalcrom, and/or a nasal steroid spray. Some show reluctance about trying these three therapies, especially those who report burning or tingling sensations or other uncomfortable or painful feelings. Because sprays are so useful in overcoming nasal congestion, please shop around for different brands of sprays with less irritation.

Monitoring Results

During the next two weeks, develop a plan to use these agents, with the aid of your doctor for prescriptions, and aggressively manage your nasal hygiene. It is essential to follow a directed plan, such as Nasalcrom two to three times per day for two weeks, then decrease to fewer doses. A large number of SDB patients need these treatments every day of the year. Plan on two to seven days to see improvements, but by two weeks at the latest, you should be near a 99 percent level of clearer nasal breathing. Thus, within seven days you could see improvements in sleep symptoms, assuming that a clearer nasal airway reduces SDB severity.

If you did not achieve an excellent nasal response, do not accept this fate. Various factors influence allergy, vasomotor rhinitis, or sinus conditions, and it is incumbent on you to further evaluate your condition. Some sinus conditions require special X-rays, such as CT scans or MRI tests, to more accurately define the full scope of the problem. A deviated nasal septum or less commonly polyps in the back of the nasal passages can be root causes of these difficulties. Again, do not hesitate to seek consultations, because failing to may prevent you from ever using advanced SDB therapies.

The NFL and Your Sleep

The next potential treatment step is very intriguing. Our research team conducted and published the first randomized, controlled study using nasal dilator strips in a group of insomnia patients. The specific nasal strip we tested was Breathe Right, often worn by football players, and we were funded by their manufacturer to conduct the study.

Before describing the results, these are the necessary disclosures:

- CNS, Inc., makers of Breathe Right, paid us only for the research and nothing else.
- CNS, Inc., did not control the study, analyze data, or write up published research reports.
- No one at our center, including myself, owns stock in CNS, Inc.

Randomized Controlled Study Design

In the study, published in the journal *Sleep and Breathing* in 2006, we researched 80 insomnia patients complaining of fairly severe middle-of-the-night awakenings resulting in more than an hour of lost sleep per night. The control group of 38 patients received general education about sleep; whereas the treatment group of 42 patients received education about potential relationships between SDB and insomnia as well as instructions on using nasal strips. We did not use polysomnography (sleep tests) to confirm SDB, but we inquired about breathing and end-organ symptoms to make presumptive diagnoses. For example, 45 of the 80 people in the study reported snoring or gasping and choking while sleeping; whereas 95 percent of them reported at least one symptom of nocturia, morning headaches, or dry mouth upon awakening.

To exclude other possible causes for awakenings, we eliminated more than 150 volunteers who also suffered other medical or psychiatric conditions, uncontrolled allergies, obesity, and other sleep disorders. We were confident that the group of participants who remained in the study exhibited a narrow scope of sleep problems, such that a relationship between their SDB and their middle-of-the-night awakenings was likely.

To rule out a bias in those who received nasal strips, we first confirmed that they had not used these devices previously, but more importantly, we asked patients whether they thought breathing problems might explain their awakenings. At the start of the study, not a single participant believed breathing could explain his or her awakenings, whereas 88 percent of the participants believed this theory was credible after being educated. The treatment group patients wore nasal strips, on average, twenty-seven of twenty-eight nights and almost always all night long.

Randomized Controlled Study Results

At the end of a month, we compared the changes in sleep between the treated group and the control group, which did not use nasal strips. The most striking results were in patients' perceptions of how much sleep problems and daytime functioning improved, although actual treatment gains by the numbers were variable. The treated patients reported large to very large improvements in insomnia and sleep quality as well as in the depth and refreshing nature of their sleep. Daytime tiredness and sleepiness showed moderate to large improvements.

Most importantly, the nasal strip users reported clear-cut changes in functioning during the day, coinciding with enhanced quality of life. These findings are impressive because quality-of-life improvements are not always reported in research using cognitive behavioral therapy (CBT) or sedatives for insomnia.

The objective numbers were less impressive, as treated patients still reported an average of two awakenings per night instead of three, whereas the control group reported barely any change in awakenings. And the number of minutes of lost sleep in the middle of the night in the treatment group improved by only twenty-four minutes, compared to twenty-one minutes in the control group. Yet these numbers may indicate successes only in terms of a sleep quantity model, whereas our perspective was to emphasize and explore sleep quality changes.

A total of twenty-three of forty-two treated patients reported marked improvements in insomnia severity, and another ten of forty-two reported some improvement, for a total of 79 percent noticing clear changes in their sleep, compared to less than a handful in the thirty-eight participants in the control group.

SLEEP ON IT
Nasal Dilator Strip Therapy

QUESTION: Nasal strips are often the next best step to attempt in treating your SDB. They are easy to use, inexpensive, and have almost no side effects. As long as you use them properly for two to four weeks, every night, you can usually clarify if they are enhancing sleep quality, which then confirms a presumptive SDB diagnosis. Are you willing to try?

COMMENT: One of the most interesting findings in the research study was that most patients who improved with nasal strips tended to report a progressive improvement the longer they wore the strips. For example, in the primary randomized control period of one month, insomnia and quality-of-life improvements had improved after two weeks of nasal strip use, but at the end of four weeks, improvements were even larger for these two sleep measures. Many treated patients reported they weren't sure how well the nasal strips helped until after wearing them for at least two weeks. Only a handful of patients were clear that nasal strips worked in the first or the second week.

Another surprising finding involved several participants who did not report improvement with nasal strips after one month, who were then persuaded to continue use. In the second or third month of regular nasal strip use, several individuals reported clearly improved sleep symptoms. Thus it may prove beneficial to use nasal dilator strips for more than one month to accurately determine whether they work, although I must caution you not to let your trial delay your need to complete a diagnostic study in a sleep lab, the details of which are covered in part seven.

——— PEARL ———
Nasal Dilator Strip Therapy Instructions

There are four steps that help you use strips effectively:

1. Size matters: you must have the correct fit for your nose.
2. Position: the strip must rest below the bridge of the nose; otherwise it will not open the nasal passages. (Feel the lower edge of the bony portion of the nose and be sure the strip rests below it.)
3. Prep work: you must wash your nose to remove oils before you place the strip, or else it will come off while you are sleeping, which means you must place the strip within a couple minutes of washing the nose.
4. Removal: you absolutely must have a plan to carefully remove the device in the morning because simply pulling it off removes or scrapes your skin. The best removal options are:
   - Remove in the shower after steam moistens the seal.
   - Using soap and water, gently and slowly leak suds under the ends of the strips to break the seal, then rub more soap against the adhesive as your fingers eventually move closer to and eventually meet at the crest of your nose.

Rarely, a person suffers irritation from the strips, which may be due to the powder in the packaging material. This problem may be solved by opening the nasal strip packaging and dropping the strip on the bathroom counter and throwing away the packaging. Then shower or wash your hands, nose, and face with soap and water, and only then place the strip.

Even small improvements in breathing and sleep are highly motivating, because they reveal that you are moving in the right direction. Individuals with severe obesity or severe psychiatric disorders have shown less improvement with nasal strips, but we have been surprised that some receive occasional good to excellent results.

25

Another Balloon to Blow Up

Assessing Your Progress

Changing sleep positions and using aggressive nasal strategies usually lead to noticeable changes within a month in a majority of troubled sleepers. If your changes were dramatic, you may want to continue your current program for another month or two, but always maintain a regular monitoring schedule to be certain you are sustaining or strengthening your gains. If changes have not been forthcoming or you know that more improvement should be expected, it's time to think more seriously about sleep-disordered breathing (SDB) and spending a night in a sleep lab.

Inflating Your Balloon

Picture a sausage-shaped balloon. Without air, it looks flat, much like a flat hose looks with no water running through it. With sufficient air for the balloon, just as with sufficient water in the hose, this flatness expands into a tube shape. The air or water pressure supplied to a balloon or a hose can be increased to maintain the tube at its full cylindrical shape, just as turning off the flow causes the tube to collapse.

The human airway operates like a collapsible tube during sleep. In sleep apnea, the tube collapses completely, which blocks any air from passing through. To reiterate, apnea is the tip of the iceberg in terms of common SDB events. Whereas it is obvious that apnea would trigger the brain to wake up to induce a new breath, can you imagine any other shape of this collapsible tube that might trigger an arousal?

In other words, how would you feel when you are choking *just a little*? There is no pleasant sensation involved in choking. We choke without any air at all, which causes the most intense panic, but we could also choke a little, which produces a little bit of panic, anxiety, or discomfort, which we wish to eliminate sooner rather than later.

Let's say the collapsible tube is half open/half closed compared to its full diameter. If this constriction caused a 50 percent reduction in airflow, then the sleep medical term would be "hypopnea." For many years, since the formal scientific discovery of SDB in the 1960s, hypopneas were not appreciated as a problem. Researchers and doctors focused on apneas, the complete cessation of breathing. Leading researchers recognized that hypopneas also caused SDB patients to suffer awakenings, arousals, and microarousals as well as fluctuations in oxygen—"desaturations" below the normal 90 percent value.

Once this connection was established, many sleep researchers and sleep medical professionals recognized that counting only the number of apneas led to incomplete diagnosis and treatment, and ultimately it severely limited our understanding of SDB.

SNOOZE FLASH
Developing Clearer Definitions of SDB

Medicare adopted a policy in the early 1980s that only required sleep labs to report the number of apneas; but worse, Medicare insisted that apneas were the only legitimate components of SDB and ignored research showing the relevance of other forms of breathing disruption. A "thirty-apnea rule" created a major barrier to treating SDB patients by narrowing the definition. Physicians thought about sleep apnea as the only form of SDB. They focused on narrow symptom presentations of this complex sleep disorder, believing that without loud snoring and daytime sleepiness, sleep apnea could not be present. This narrow perspective haunted the field of sleep medicine for two decades, yet many sleep professionals never gave up the cause, and in 2001, Medicare adopted a new rule including hypopneas in the SDB definition.

Chart 4. Sleep-Disordered Breathing Events

A. Normal Breathing

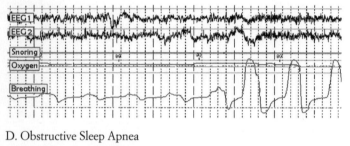

B. Upper Airway Resistance

C. Hypopnea

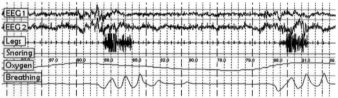

D. Obstructive Sleep Apnea

All graphs span sixty seconds, and the upper portion of the breathing tracing represents inspiration and the lower half represents expiration. The breathing tracings start with normal, then show progressive worsening. Note that snoring is *absent* in all panels. Observe the changes, both subtle and large, in oxygenation levels. (A). Normal Breathing. The upper curve looks symmetrical, but the lower curve tapers off to a flat line signifying the natural pause in exhalation that occurs prior to restarting inhalation. Note how oxygen remains steady at 95 percent. (B). Upper Airway Resistance. The very top of the inspiratory curve is cutoff or notched, indicating a restriction in airflow that eventually leads to an arousal and then two large, normal breaths (note how the brain waves speed up just before better breathing). Oxygen stays constant at 93 percent throughout. (C.) Hypopnea. The airflow signal is now radically depressed but still shows air movement. Oxygen fluctuates in a narrow range between 88 and 90 percent. (D). Obstructive Sleep Apnea. The airflow signal shows a flat line (no air movement), followed by an arousal, a leg jerk just after the arousal, and three quick breaths, and then another apnea followed by the same cycle. Notice the wide fluctuations in oxygenation between 78 and 91 percent. The leg jerk may be an arousal due to the apnea.

Little Bad Breaths

I wish this Medicare tale were the end of a story in which everyone slept happily ever after, but recall that even a little choking is still choking. As research continued, a phenomenal pioneer, Dr. Christian Guilleminault, discovered subtle forms of breathing disturbance. He demonstrated that these subtle forms of choking or collapsing of the airway also caused the brain to speed up and arouse or awaken the sleeper. He called this version of SDB "upper airway resistance syndrome" (UARS), implying that the tube might collapse only a tiny bit or not at all, but for various reasons, airflow encountered resistance in passing through the nose or oral airways.

You can see pictures of all these different types of breathing events in the chart on page 240.

Dr. Guilleminault discovered that patients, particularly women and children, could suffer from SDB without a single apnea or hypopnea. Instead, the patient endured so many upper airway resistance events that she presented with similar symptoms of sleep fragmentation seen in sleep apnea patients. In these UARS patients, SDB could be diagnosed and treated as if they had sleep apnea. In 1995 Dr. Guilleminault reported on a large sample of women who suffered almost exclusively from upper airway resistance events, and he demonstrated that aggressive SDB therapy not only reversed their daytime sleepiness but also decreased or eliminated their trips to the bathroom at night. In this particular study, he also described women with SDB who did not snore.

Dr. Guilleminault, who I had the pleasure and grand fortune of training under for three months in 1993 at Stanford University Sleep Disorders Center, did not find great receptivity to his ideas, which is not surprising for someone so far ahead on the cutting edge of science. Remarkably, Dr. Guilleminault made this discovery of upper airway resistance in the late 1970s while studying children with SDB. Yet, now more than a quarter century later, Medicare and a host of insurance carriers as well as many medical professionals outside the field of sleep medicine have not formally recognized the role of UARS. Regrettably, some of these institutions and physicians seem to be developing their judgments without any real-world, clinical sleep medicine experiences or expertise.

UARS Pearls

Depending on the sleep center at which you seek treatment, some sleep physicians will not test for upper airway resistance because of their frustrations in dealing with these insurance carriers. This issue is highly problematic, because sleep doctors must struggle to help the patient the best way possible, but some insurance companies laid down rules, often in lockstep with Medicare, that prevent prescribing appropriate treatment.

This snafu may prove critical to your treatment, because it seems that many insomnia patients suffer from upper airway resistance events. Remarkably, most sleep research on insomnia or psychiatric patients has ignored upper airway resistance. This lack of attention to breathing in general and the precision of breathing disruption in particular have caused tremendous confusion in our understanding of sleep problems in patients with insomnia or mental health complaints.

At our sleep research institute, we conducted the first study to examine upper airway resistance in psychiatric patients, which was published in the journal of *Biological Psychiatry* in 2001. In a small sample of crime victims with posttraumatic stress symptoms who were seeking help for insomnia, we diagnosed forty of forty-four patients with SDB. The data corroborated the points above, showing that it is essential to count all types of SDB breathing events to properly make a diagnosis and assess severity level. In our study, using apneas, hypopneas, and upper airway resistance events, the average crime victim experienced nearly forty disruptive breathings per hour or, on average, more than two hundred arousals or awakenings due to SDB in just one night.

Chicken or Egg?

This research raises the tantalizing question about the potentially high rates of SDB in mental health patients. In our studies, we have proposed two theories that revolve around the common findings of insomnia and emotional distress in psychiatric patients. First, an enormous number of patients with mental disorders suffer from unwanted bouts of sleeplessness that plague the individual for years. As it turns out, insomnia itself seems to increase your risk for SDB, because insomnia causes you to spend too much time in lighter sleep, such as stage 1 NREM. In this lighter stage, your breathing is more susceptible to disruption from apneas, hypopneas, or UARS events. Thus, while the mental health patient might start out with insomnia and no SDB, it's possible that SDB develops over a period of persistently fragmented sleep.

We also speculate that emotional distress, particularly anxiety, directly impacts the human airway, causing some type of tension or restriction. In other words, we wonder whether a person can develop UARS, as one example, just by being nervous for so long that it adversely influences breathing.

Eventually, changes caused by insomnia and distress may foster the clinical emergence of sleep-disordered breathing, particularly in the form of UARS. We have worked with many trauma survivors who reported no sleep problems prior to a traumatic event. Then posttrauma, they developed nightmares and insomnia, which were never treated. Sleep got progressively worse, and eventually they were tested and found to have SDB. It would be very interesting to find out how early in the course of their sleep problems they actually developed the first signs of SDB. And, for these reasons, we are much more aggressive now in recommending sleep testing as early as possible for someone with insomnia.

SNOOZE FLASH

The Respiratory Threat Matrix Model of Chronic Insomnia: A Special Mind-Body Sleep Theory

Dovetailing with these interesting questions is another theory we propose that alleges SDB not only causes awakenings at night, but SDB also prevents you from falling asleep at bedtime or returning to sleep if awakened at night.

It's easy to see how an SDB event awakens you. If the struggle for a good breath lasts too long, and your mind starts churning away, you soon find yourself fully awake. The main breathing disruption occurred first, but you don't remember it. You blame racing thoughts and ruminations for the awakening and the inability to return to sleep.

In this SDB two-step (struggle for breath, racing thoughts), which element is more intense: a minisuffocation or your racing thoughts? The bet here is on breathing disruption as the more nerve-racking and fraught with more intensely unpleasant feelings. Ruminations may be bothersome, but an SDB event is more immediate and threatening. Imagine a pillow placed on your face as you fall asleep. The pillow causes minisuffocations, so you knock it off, but somehow it gets replaced again and again. This analogy mirrors SDB events. You would never know about the pillow, but still, wouldn't you hesitate about going to sleep? Wouldn't some anxiety arise when you walk in the bedroom and a lot more anxiety when you climb into bed?

Here's the punch line that often knocks sleep patients into an entirely new orbit. What if you happen to be a heckuva lot smarter (which I am quite certain of) about your sleep problems than you first thought? What if you are so smart you decide it's a lot safer to stay awake instead of going to or returning to sleep? What if you develop the instinct that you really do not want to be asleep, because being awake clearly prevents breathing events and feelings of suffocation?

What if you "choose" not to sleep? If you made that "choice," what's the fastest, most reliable way to keep yourself awake? You got it: stir up enough racing thoughts and ruminations to stay awake and not have another SDB event. Sounds unbelievable, doesn't it?

Although it's just a theory we've been working on at our research institute, numerous SDB patients report a decrease in racing thoughts and ruminations just by treating their breathing condition. Several have called it a mini-miracle, because they pursued no other therapies, no medications or psychological treatments whatsoever. They simply used a breathing mask treatment at bedtime, and their minds went to sleep without further ado. Adding to their convictions, they reported a newfound capacity to roll over and return to sleep without hesitation in the middle of the night. Without any prompting, these SDB patients reported these phenomenal changes in their racing thoughts and ruminations and linked the changes to SDB therapy.

The most astonished and astonishing patients were those suffering from severe sleep onset insomnia. At bedtime they required one to two hours to fall asleep, and most used sleeping pills. Some of these patients declared that SDB treatment completely eliminated their racing thoughts and ruminations, not to mention their need for sleeping pills, because they could fall asleep in less than ten minutes.

In many of these severe insomnia patients who were tested in our sleep lab, we noticed a pattern of frequent breathing irregularities—while awake—as they tried unsuccessfully to fall asleep. None of them were aware of any breathing difficulties while awake or asleep. Yet, just by replacing their "bad breaths" with good breaths by using positive airway pressure (PAP) therapy as they attempted to sleep, their minds appeared to replace their racing thoughts with the *Wave of Sleepiness*.

So, what happened? Did PAP therapy simply produce a general relaxation response by stabilizing breathing, or did PAP therapy eliminate the possible fear of suffocation, which eliminated the "need" for racing thoughts? We don't know, but of greater interest, many of these patients reported that their daytime anxiety levels also decreased once they regularly used PAP therapy.

Make Every Bad Breath Count

When SDB is tested in the sleep lab, the correct way, as required by the American Academy of Sleep Medicine, is to count all SDB events. The test results add up apneas, hypopneas, and upper airway resistance events. The total number of events is then divided by the total number of hours slept. If a person suffered 210 breathing events during 7 hours of sleep, then the quotient of these numbers (210 events ÷ 7 hours) equals 30 events per hour. This number is called the Respiratory Disturbance Index, or RDI, which equals 30 in the example.

RDI levels are frequently described in the following ways:

- Mild SDB = RDI between 5 and 20 events per hour.
- Moderate SDB = RDI between 20 and 40 events per hour.
- Severe SDB = RDI greater than 40 events per hour.

In our study of crime victims, if we counted only apneas and hypopneas and *not* upper airway resistance events, then the RDI of these trauma survivors would have been only about 10 events per hour, equivalent to mild cases. When we added in the upper airway resistance events, the RDI skyrocketed to an average of nearly 40 events per hour, a much more severe condition. When you decide to undergo a sleep test, be sure to find a lab that gives the full RDI.

Central Apneas

Last, while most breathing disruption is caused by different forms of obstruction or resistance, some patients, particularly those with medical conditions of the heart, lung, or brain systems, suffer "central" events caused by malfunctions in the central nervous system in those portions of the brain that control respiratory drive. Central events are sometimes related to changes in oxygen and carbon dioxide concentrations. When higher or lower concentrations of these gases are delivered by the blood supply to the critical breathing centers in the brain, they may cause a breathing switch to momentarily pause.

In a central event, you'll see that neither the chest nor the abdomen are moving as they normally would when trying to overcome an obstruction. Instead, there is no motion, because the brain has signaled the body to stop breathing. As you may discover, central apnea sometimes occurs in a patient who, while attempting to use positive airway pressure (PAP) therapy, develops a startle response to the pressurized airflow coming in, then momentarily stops breathing. Sleep technologists and sleep specialists must make more concerted efforts to help patients resolve central apnea, from whatever causes.

SLEEP ON IT
Oxygen Checkup

QUESTION: As a final step in your diagnostic assessments, you should also evaluate whether SDB influences other chronic illnesses you may suffer from. Have you discussed the potential for an SDB diagnosis with your doctor, and have you discussed the relationships between SDB and other ailments from which you suffer?

COMMENT: Normal sleepers breathe with a consistency that yields stable oxygen levels. If you tracked the oxygen sensor of a normal sleeper, you see an unwavering signal. The oxygen levels might be 95 percent for thirty continuous seconds or sixty continuous seconds or several minutes. SDB patients suffer oxygen fluctuations; the level frequently drops a few percentage points or more when breathing is disrupted, then returns to a consistent level after an arousal or awakening. If you start at 95 percent, it could drop to 94 percent, 92 percent, or 90 percent, all in thirty seconds or less. The signal can fluctuate up and down in this narrow range all night.

For patients with severe SDB, oxygen desaturates below the normal level of 90 percent into damaging ranges of 80 percent or 70 percent. In the most severe forms of sleep apnea, a patient drops his oxygen level into life-threatening ranges below 70 percent, which could produce short- and long-term serious damage to the heart and brain, and which triggers dangerous cardiac arrhythmias (heart rhythm disturbances).

Interference with the body's natural, highly stable oxygen baseline during sleep and related sleep fragmentation clearly translates into poor health. For example, in normal sleep, the body's natural recuperative processes lower blood pressure for much of the night, a process called "dipping," which rests the cardiovascular system. However, in SDB patients suffering either sleep fragmentation or oxygen fluctuation, "dipping" disappears, and blood pressure remains at higher levels than expected during the night. Remarkably, aggressive treatment of SDB restores dipping and lowers blood pressure in some patients. If SDB affects such an intricate physiological process such as blood pressure, what else might it affect during the night as well as during the day?

> **SNOOZE FLASH**
>
> ### SDB Is More Than Just a Sleep Disorder
>
> Why would SDB affect so many different aspects of mental and physical health?
>
> The answer is simple: **SDB is a multisystem disease** that affects nearly every major system of the body. The reason why SDB has such global influence goes beyond sleep fragmentation and oxygenation desaturations. Worse, SDB promotes **oxidative stress**, a crucial biochemical pathway in which various harmful biomolecules circulate through the body, causing cell damage or outright destruction.
>
> Oxidative stress is the pathway through which cigarette smoking, heart disease, and various infectious diseases causes inflammation in tissues and organs, leading to poorer functioning. Oxidative stress also has been linked to aging, and there is no question that SDB contributes adversely to the aging process, which brings up a fact you won't soon forget: Nearly all people who successfully treat their SDB will find that their family, friends, or coworkers will comment about how much healthier or younger they look within weeks of starting the treatment.
>
> Slowly but surely, SDB is a sleeping sickness that literally sleeps you older and older, robbing you of your mental and physical health. Now, more than ever, you need to fight back and regain your health by aggressively targeting this monster so you can have *Sound Sleep* night after night.

─────── PEARL ───────

SDB Impact on the Rest of Your Health

Here are several important considerations that would be in your best interests to evaluate if applicable as you continue your efforts to determine whether you suffer from SDB. If you suffer from:

- high blood pressure, an aggressive SDB treatment may result in a noticeable lowering of pressure, which sometimes requires a reduction in blood pressure medication.
- a form of diabetes known as insulin resistance, your glucose control may improve following aggressive SDB treatment.

- heart disease in the form of congestive heart failure, heart attacks, or heart rhythm disturbances, your risks for the worsening of these heart problems may decrease with aggressive SDB treatment.
- chronic or intermittent bouts of depression, aggressive SDB treatment may mitigate the depression, which in turn may require an adjustment of antidepressant medication.
- fibromyalgia or other chronic pain symptoms or fatigue, any of which might be worsened by a sleep disorder, aggressive SDB treatment is likely to reduce some of these symptoms.
- alcoholism, drug abuse, or addiction problems, aggressive SDB treatment will reduce fatigue or sleepiness, which might then decrease urges to use such substances.

PART SEVEN

HIGH-TECH SLEEP SOLUTIONS

Custom-Tailored Sleep Treatment

A Cure Is Just around the Corner

Remember that magic sleep wand we've talked about? Now you're going to discover a truly magic sleep machine. It's not so difficult to use (I use one every night, all night long), although learning to use one takes time and effort. And there are thousands of sleep medical centers in the United States offering services to help you do just that.

The bulk of this section covers how to work in your local area with sleep medicine specialists as well as the suppliers of the breathing device equipment.

There's also a chapter on leg movement disorders and then a final chapter on future pathways and resources to consider in your quest for *Sound Sleep*, if you are not satisfied with the results so far.

For many, this part of the book is best read in preparation to visiting a sleep medical center or during your work with an area sleep specialist.

26

Acing Your Sleep Test

A Night in the Lab

We live in an extraordinary age of technology in which we now easily measure a vast array of physiological functions of the human body, such as blood sugar, bone density, heart rhythms, lung volumes, blood pressure, diameter of the coronary arteries, heart pumping efficiency, and so on. Now we can measure sleep breathing with much precision.

To undergo this test, however, you would be asked to do an odd thing: spend a night in a sleep lab, hooked up to nearly twenty different sensors, during which a technician watches you all night long through an infrared camera that feeds to a television monitor, and have the technician enter your bedroom several times during the night to check on your sensors, to confirm your snoring, mouth breathing, body position, and any other unusual movements or noises you might make . . . and all this activity occurs while you are supposedly sleeping!

Although what we learn about your sleep in the lab proves so insightful and exciting—enough to take your breath away—one significant obstacle might hamper your efforts to schedule a test: getting you to agree to spend the night in the lab!

Unequivocally, your emotions are the most important factors determining whether:

- you spend a night in the lab;
- you actually sleep in the lab;
- you become motivated by the information discovered in the lab.

The single greatest barrier to the lab is your emotional response to it or related feelings about the likelihood of suffering sleep-disordered breathing (SDB). Embarrassment, shame, guilt, fear, anxiety, pain, or discomfort clearly stall people's efforts. A large number of SDB sufferers who wish to avoid these emotional responses insist that the whole matter is a big inconvenience and block out their deeper concerns.

Any discussion to effectively motivate you to undergo sleep testing and to consider advanced SDB treatments must address your emotional responses, all of which takes time. But you have the tools now to work through your emotional concerns and forge ahead.

How do you feel about sleeping in a lab? Wouldn't you like to know the number of breathing events in your Respiratory Disturbance Index (RDI)?

Sleep Centers and Sleep Specialists

Most sleep specialists have trained in pulmonary medicine. Others have backgrounds in internal medicine, family medicine, pediatrics, and neurology, and a smaller proportion trained first in psychiatry or psychology. The good news in working with a board-certified sleep specialist is that you are in good hands for matters strictly concerning your sleep; however, only a small proportion of these doctors practice in a mind-body medicine style consistent with all components of Sleep Dynamic Therapy (SDT). Few have specific training in cognitive-behavioral, imagery, or emotional processing therapies.

A sleep doctor's experience largely depends on the types of patients seen and how regularly he or she sees complex patients. Even if a physician develops a great deal of expertise in helping sleep patients overcome emotional responses to sleep disorders, most sleep physicians work in the world of managed scare, where the goal is to ration health-care resources as well as to restrict time spent between doctor and patient. We believe that a large proportion of troubled sleepers need more time to address emotional concerns about and barriers to advanced SDB therapies, which means working through these emotions as much as possible before you ever visit a sleep doctor.

Making matters potentially more problematic, many sleep medical facilities are sleep labs only, without clinical operations. They usually have a board-certified sleep doctor reading and interpreting sleep studies, but you are not offered the chance to meet with this doctor. The sleep test information is sent back to your referring physician, who usually has negligible training in sleep medicine. Depending on this physician's interests and experience, he or she may provide you with a little or a lot of support and technical supervision in managing your SDB treatment. Your best overall care plan, in the minds of board-certified sleep physicians, involves the potential to consult a sleep specialist. Then again, some areas have limited sleep medical resources, and a sleep lab may be the only pathway available.

A bright spot on the horizon is the new subspecialty within our field known as Behavioral Sleep Medicine. This branch advances the use of cognitive-behavioral strategies to treat sleep disorders. Sleep specialists with training, experience, or certification in Behavioral Sleep Medicine bring a much-needed component into the clinics, because these professionals use advanced insomnia strategies.

To find a sleep center to accommodate your needs, many factors must be considered. If you live in or near a large metropolitan area, you have more options and can scout around.

Sleeping Around

The secret to a successful night at the sleep lab boils down to two things:

1. effective sleep technologists who attend to your needs;
2. advanced technology to measure your sleep breathing.

Polysomnography technologists—the sleep techs who spend the night with you—hook you up to sensors and monitor your sleep. These professionals are the backbone of any sleep disorders center. Without competent, reliable, trustworthy, compassionate, empathetic, and communicative sleep techs, a sleep lab or sleep center develops a poor reputation, which cannot be overcome by the most superlative physicians and other daytime sleep center staff. You must spend the night with this tech, and you deserve and require a professional who understands this work and cares about patients. This technologist must attach sensors to your body while you are in pajamas or less, and this tech frequently enters your bedroom, both while you are asleep and awake, to make adjustments and observations and to ensure that the data collected meet appropriate standards.

Tech training is highly variable and depends on the mix of patients seen at the particular sleep center at which training occurs. Some centers have no specific training for managing posttraumatic stress disorder (PTSD) patients or other psychiatric patients in need of sleep studies. This is unfortunate, because these patients are increasingly referred to sleep centers. Without attending to their special needs, many centers experience more "no-shows" for testing or a greater number of individuals who leave before the test is completed, because these patients' nerves fray quickly, and then they bolt in the middle of the night.

Planning ahead may help you find the best sleep center.

Selecting a Center

There is no easy way to evaluate sleep labs or centers beforehand. If you are in an outlying area, your local sleep lab is a reasonable option. If you have a choice, inquire about five things

1. Do they use a technology to measure upper airway resistance?
2. Do they score upper airway resistance syndrome (UARS) and include it in the RDI?
3. If your insurance company battles you on a UARS diagnosis, will the sleep center support you?
4. Do they offer daytime breathing mask desensitization programs to try out the mask for thirty to sixty minutes?
5. Will they review test results on a computer screen to demonstrate to you the highlights of your sleep disorder?

Centers and labs with these attributes are likely to be more advanced facilities that appreciate essentials of a mind-body approach. You may have personal preferences or requests; for example, Do they have a refrigerator if you need a snack before bedtime or in the middle of the night? What are the mattresses like? These types of concerns are almost always well attended to by every sleep center and sleep lab operation. For just about anything you can think of, the facilities have already experienced it enough times to install a system to accommodate such needs or concerns.

Frustrations and concerns arise at or after testing for other reasons:

- Will you have any choice in the type of study scheduled?
- What if the sleep tech is not helpful or communicative during the test night?

- How long will it take to get the results back?
- Will you get to see a doctor?

Types of Sleep Studies

Some sleep centers conduct split-night protocols, during which the first half of the night diagnoses SDB, and the second half tests out the positive airway pressure (PAP) breathing mask to determine your response and best pressures. PAP is the air compressor that pushes air through a tube connected to a mask over your nose or mouth or both, which then keeps your airway pinned open. Many centers schedule split-night protocols, because they believe this model is efficient and saves money. We concur with this view when the patient is a classic sleep apnea patient without complications—that is, they do not suffer from insomnia and mental health factors, such as trauma history, claustrophobia, or other mental health disorders. As such, our center orders a split-night protocol in less than 10 percent of patients, because we see few patients without these complexities. We

SNOOZE FLASH

Getting Hooked

When hooked up in the lab, you have sensors or leads all over your body to monitor physiological signs of sleep, breathing, movements, and so on, including:

- electroencephalographic (EEG) leads to measure brain waves awake and asleep;
- eye leads to measure eye movements to determine REM sleep;
- airflow sensors to measure nasal breathing and mouth breathing;
- chin sensor to measure changes in muscle tension and teeth grinding;
- a snore sensor, which may be placed on your neck;
- EKG leads to monitor your heart;
- chest and abdominal bands to measure movement of chest and abdomen during breathing;
- leg sensors to measure leg movements;
- a finger or other probe measuring oxygen or carbon dioxide.

Bring a camera and get a photo. Your kids or friends will love it.

suspect that many sleep centers have a high proportion of patients with these complexities, but they choose split-night protocols anyway, which often leads to poor results.

If you have a choice, we encourage a diagnostic study, not a split night for your first test. A diagnostic study makes things simpler and removes any tension about using the mask before you are ready. It also facilitates your communication with the sleep tech, who may feel apprehensive in splitting a study with someone with insomnia or mental health problems. If, however, you cannot stand the idea of having two sleep studies, then the split-night protocol might get it all done in one night.

If the tech proves noncommunicative or nonsupportive, you can still get good data, but you may want to request a different tech for your next study when trying the breathing mask.

Most centers operate with you seeing the sleep physician first, then appropriate tests are ordered, but at a lab you just get the test done. After a diagnostic test, the information is relayed to the pertinent doctor, who decides about the need for further testing with PAP therapy. In some settings the sleep doctor may see you in person to discuss the next steps, phone you to discuss how to proceed, or simply make the recommendation for you and your referring doctor to follow. For example, a sleep lab may have no option for you to see the sleep physician, or you may have to travel far to actually meet a sleep physician.

The range of experience is quite wide, so ask questions to properly plan.

Advanced Technologies

To get the most out of your sleep test, you want to ensure that breathing is measured effectively and precisely. An older technology known as "thermistors" measured airflow indirectly by monitoring the changes in temperature between air coming in (colder) and air going out (warmer); the temperature differential estimates the collapsibility of the tube. The problem with a thermistor is that it's slow and indirect and cannot capture actual respiration. It's a bit like using a ruler with only inches marked off, when you need something that measures an eighth or a sixteenth of an inch, too. If you select a lab that uses only thermistors, they might miss a fair amount of information about SDB.

Many sleep labs are switching to or adding a newer technology, known as the "pressure transducer," which directly measures airflow. This device detects subtle forms of breathing disruption—the upper airway resistance events. Apnea still appears as a flat line, indicating the absence of breathing; hypopneas show about a 50 percent reduction in airflow; and the pressure transducer signal shows a "flattening" or "scooping" at the top of inspiration (or expiration for some patients), coinciding with UARS. As in chart 4, page 240, you can follow this resistance in breathing to its common conclusion—a microarousal, an arousal, or an awakening. You see the flattened breaths marching out in a pattern, at the end of which the brain speeds up to breathe better. The signal then shows normal breaths; the person falls back asleep and starts again with flattening or scooping. The cycle is repeated hundreds of times per night in UARS patients.

SLEEP ON IT
Spend Your Sleep Wisely

QUESTION: Most people with a worried or anxious mind-set imagine that a lot will go wrong during their sleep test, such as not finding out what's really going on with their sleep, because they will not sleep the same way as at home. Are you worried that something won't show up?

COMMENT: The remarkable thing about sleeping in the lab is that if you have a breathing disorder, it almost always shows up. No matter what complicating circumstances you imagine to interfere with the test, your anticipated problem rarely materializes.

Take one of the worst-case scenarios in which the troubled sleeper sleeps for only sixty minutes during the night and stays awake for another six, seven, eight, or nine hours. In this situation, most people not only demonstrate the breathing problem during the sixty minutes, if they really have it, but also they demonstrate a lot of interesting data during the waking portion. Many of these individuals show irregular breathing patterns while awake, and these breathing disruptions frequently indicate a clear obstacle to falling asleep. In many circumstances, even a bad night in the lab still yields enough data to enable a sleep physician to arrive at or come extremely close to making a diagnosis.

Because problematic sleepers tend to worry, they think they can gauge what will happen with their sleep in the lab, but as you recall, you are the least reliable witness to know what goes on during your sleep. Even if you never slept at all—which happens so rarely that most sleep centers don't see it once during a whole year of operation—we still gather relevant information about breathing, leg movements, or other physical factors affecting sleep.

——— PEARL ———
A One-Night Stand Worth Taking

If you are worried about waking up at night in the lab, keep these pointers in mind:

- First and foremost, don't freak out! Virtually anyone who undergoes a sleep test will awaken at various points in the night and still get back to sleep.
- For one or two nights before the sleep test, consider restricting your sleep at home by one hour each night, so you come for your test with some extra sleepiness.
- Actively plan to bring to the lab something you now use to overcome awakenings; focus on relaxation and entertainment techniques, not on productivity.
- Develop a specific imagery protocol for the sleep lab. If possible, visit lab bedrooms beforehand. Then, at home, picture yourself sleeping there. Otherwise, develop imagery of a one-night vacation during which you have no responsibilities.
- Develop a specific imagery tool for a middle-of-the-night awakening. Bring a picture book that helps you return to sleep.
- If you take medications day or night, we ask patients to stick with those meds as usual, as do most sleep centers or labs.
- Never underestimate the power of your emotional processing skills. Anxiety is the most likely emotion to interfere with your sleep. Many people develop performance anxiety about sleeping in the lab. They are also nervous about sleeping in front of a stranger or under an infrared camera. Emotions always win, so pay close attention to your feelings as you prepare.

A decent sleep lab experience can be thwarted by a poor sleep tech. Although poor sleep technologists' skill levels may be weak due to inadequate training and experience, we don't find many noncommunicative types who enter this field. Most individuals are interested in caring for patients. A sizable number of sleep techs recognize their own sleep problems and use PAP breathing masks, which makes them ideally suited to help you. If you find yourself trying to sleep in an unsupportive environment, then consider these pointers:

- Foremost, be honest with yourself about the level of anxiety that might crop up in the lab. An unsupportive or untrained sleep tech is not likely to talk you down. If you are worried about high anxiety and lack confidence in your emotional processing skills, then by all means develop a fallback medication plan with the sleep physician. This might include a prescription sedative or over-the-counter aid, which in general rarely interferes with study results with respect to SDB.
- Don't take things personally, but don't take any unprofessional treatment. Most labs have one tech for every two patients, and some have one tech for three patients. The tech also needs to eat during the night and use the bathroom. Many doze off at times for a few minutes, even though napping is inappropriate and unethical behavior. They are human, and depending on their mood and emotional processing skills, you could get a great tech, but one who is also sleep-deprived from working too many night shifts in a row or from burning the candle at both ends by not even sleeping sufficiently during the day. This job is what they were trained for and paid for. If they act discourteously, you should clearly express your concerns as diplomatically as possible, because the last thing you want is to stew all night about how frustrated or angry you are due to the sleep tech's poor behavior.
- Last, certain trauma survivors, especially veterans and sexual assault survivors, are so nervous about what might happen in the lab at night, as they have so much trouble at night anyway, that they might be better off sleeping in the lab during the daytime, even if the study turns out to be shorter. Even though the test may not be as thorough, it proves sufficient to make a diagnosis, and the troubled sleeper finds the experience much less anxiety-producing. However, many sleep centers and labs do not routinely offer a daytime test.

27

A Return to the Lab

Show Me the Results

If you went to an emergency room with a broken leg, do you imagine the doctor would show you the actual break on the X-ray film? The sleep facilities that treat you should appreciate the importance of your eyes taking in and digesting health information. Not only is seeing believing, but also the images give you confidence in moving forward on your next treatment decisions.

We educate our patients by showing them the actual sleep study. This session takes less than ten minutes or more than an hour. In more than 50 percent of lab testing situations, we show patients a few pertinent images from their study the very morning they arise from bed. Although we would like to use this protocol with every patient, logistical issues such as work and children's school schedules often prevent everyone from seeing their pictures that morning, so we bring them back for another appointment or at their next test to review their results.

These sessions do not pin down the diagnosis, which can be completed only by the sleep physician. The purpose is to enhance the patient's momentum. Most sleep-disordered breathing (SDB) patients show obvious breathing events. Some show snoring, when they thought they did not snore. When the patients walk out the door and the last impression they recall is the image of an apnea, hypopnea, or UARS event, they are more interested and motivated in pursuing the next therapeutic steps.

Return Engagement

Returning to the lab a second time seems like a royal pain, but it also could prove the single step that completely changes your perspective about sleep problems, and it just might change the direction of your life. The breathing mask treatment consists of using a mask to apply positive airway pressure—PAP therapy. This pressure prevents the collapsible tube of your airway from closing down, and by keeping it open and stable, your mind-body no longer conspires to wake you up hundreds of times during the night.

The pressure is just air, not oxygen, except for severe SDB cases. This pressure sensation is present when you breathe in and out. With just one night of PAP therapy, if you adapt to it, then you wake up in the morning and immediately recognize the difference between *Poor Sleep Quality* and *Sound Sleep*.

Chart 5 on the following page shows normal breathing in a patient using PAP therapy. This normalized airflow means that the apneas, hypopneas, and upper airway resistance events have been eliminated. However, as you'll see on the chart and learn in this chapter and the next, sleep movements or other types of arousals many still interfere with your sleep, even if your breathing is normal.

If you are itching for the split-night pathway, because you want to get it all done in one night, then many sleep centers offer this test. If you are highly motivated and anticipate no anxiety, fear, embarrassment, shame, discomfort, or pain related to the mask or the pressure, then go for it. However, please consider a few advantages to a second study in the lab with a full night of PAP therapy using the breathing mask:

- You feel less fear or anxiety about adapting, because you use it the whole night.
- You obtain more REM sleep, the most critical sleep stage to test.
- You obtain more supine sleep, the most critical position to test.
- Combining the last two points means that you test more supine REM sleep, wherein SDB is more intense and needs higher pressures.
- You gain more time to try out different masks for fitting and comfort; chinstraps if you mouth-breathe; and PAP delivery systems, which may be the most critical part of adaptation.

To decide the test for your needs, you want to return to your imagery and emotional processing skills to examine the following issues:

Chart 5. Normalized Breathing with Bilevel PAP Therapy

A. Normal Breathing

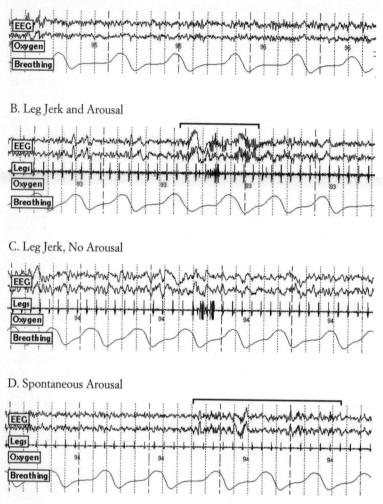

B. Leg Jerk and Arousal

C. Leg Jerk, No Arousal

D. Spontaneous Arousal

Each graph spans thirty seconds. Breathing was normalized on positive airway pressure (PAP) therapy, the bilevel type, in all four graphics. (A). Normal Breathing. Oxygen is very stable, and brain waves show no arousals. When an SDB patient achieves this optimal response all night, it may reduce or eliminate insomnia. (B). Leg Jerk with Arousal. Despite normal breathing, the patient suffers a leg jerk with an arousal. Leg jerks may cause more sleep fragmentation or prevent an optimal response to PAP therapy. (C). Leg Jerk, No Arousal. This leg jerk does not speed up brain waves, and it may or may not impact sleep quality. SDB patients on antidepressants frequently show this pattern. (D). Spontaneous Arousal. Breathing, oxygenation, and leg channels are normal, yet brain waves still speed up spontaneously. Spontaneous arousals arise in everyone at various rates, but insomniacs may show more of these arousals before or after using PAP therapy.

- Do you have claustrophobia or claustrophobic-like anxieties or fears about putting a mask on your face to help you breathe?

   The breathing mask might easily trigger anxiety and fear among susceptible sleepers.
- Do you have concerns about discomfort or pain, which might be impossible to tolerate when placing something on your face?

   The idea of sleeping with a mask on your face may be a nonstarter. For some, it worsens sleep at first, sometimes for weeks, due to the foreignness of the mask.
- Do you have relationship conflicts or personal beliefs that might trigger embarrassment, shame, or guilt about using a mask?

   Many people imagine that wearing a breathing mask ends their sex life. Others feel flawed, the way a diabetic may feel about injecting insulin. In our clinical experience, embarrassment is the single greatest barrier to the use of the breathing mask.

Turning Things Around

Three factors trigger the feelings and emotions described above:

1. the sensations of wearing the mask on your face;
2. the sensations of the pressurized air in your nose or mouth;
3. the impact of the whole experience on yourself or your relationships.

Sleep Dynamic Therapy (SDT) was developed as a mind-body program based on our experience that the overwhelming majority of troubled sleepers benefit from a breathing device. To use a mask, psychological treatments are needed to accept and utilize this unusual physiological treatment. Now is the time to use every tool to overcome unpleasant thoughts, feelings, and images triggered by these barriers.

It does not necessarily matter where you start, but you must understand that it is an adaptation process that could take days, weeks, months, or a year to fully accept and then use PAP therapy every night. That's right—one year for a few people—so patience is a big virtue, and given that you have likely suffered sleep disturbances and SDB for years or decades, count yourself among the lucky if you integrate the whole experience in a month.

The most important first step is getting a good start. Research shows that if you have a bad start—say, in the first four days of trying PAP therapy at home—there's a high probability you'll scrap the whole thing.

Clearly, the most important first step is to have a productive night in the lab the first time you use PAP therapy. Notice I didn't say a great night. A productive night means:

- You slept for a few consecutive hours with the mask in place.
- The technologist tested various pressure levels and PAP delivery systems to see what you might start with at home.
- You feel different in the morning or the next afternoon, which means your sleep quality improved overnight.
- The experience was not traumatizing, painful, or uncomfortable, so you can still imagine trying PAP therapy at home.

In a Day's Work

One of the most reliable preparations for this first night in the lab is not to go anywhere near the lab . . . at night. Under apt circumstances, visit a center some time before your test, to undergo a desensitization and fitting procedure. Many centers provide these steps the night of the study before the actual test. This timing is pragmatic, but it may not prepare you for a full-night PAP titration study. Take note of factors most relevant to your circumstances and preferences as you read about these possible desensitization steps.

Discomfort and Pain. You may have trepidation just about putting this thing on your face. The goal is to find a comfortable mask before you ever feel the pressure. The revolution in mask technology has made it possible for almost everyone to find a comfortable mask. If the sleep center has a limited supply of styles, shop for another mask after your first PAP test. I have used the Puritan Bennett Breeze nasal pillows mask for years, because it forms an arc over my narrow facial structure, and nothing presses onto my face except the little nasal prong-like structures that fit comfortably in my nostrils. If any part of a mask causes pain, you are unlikely to adapt to PAP therapy. A mask may cause pain due to a poor fit, a wrong size, or if it's worn the wrong way. Don't settle for pain; assume it needs to be fixed.

Anxiety and Fear. Placing a mask on your face, over your nose, or over your mouth and nose would be fine if you're scuba diving. (By the way, scuba divers adapt to breathing masks as fast as or faster than anyone. So you could learn to scuba dive first, and then try PAP therapy.) Some patients rip the mask off their faces the instant the straps are applied to keep it in place. So don't strap the mask on at first; just hold it up to your face with your own hands.

Once a patient expresses comfort with a mask, we try PAP therapy, preferably in the sitting position first with the mask strapped or unstrapped. Either way is fine, but if anxiety and fear rise, don't strap it on right away. The anxiety and fear trigger claustrophobic or panic responses in some. This type of response is usually learned early in life. Most poor sleepers who worry about claustrophobia also report at least one of the following events at a young age:

- near-drowning;
- pillows stuffed tightly over the face by siblings;
- locked in a closet as a prank;
- suffocated during a pile-on with other kids.

Regardless of why these experiences occurred, they were somewhat to greatly traumatizing. Most claustrophobic patients detect something in the past that triggered the phobia, but they can overcome this problem through similar desensitization steps as we are discussing here.

Red in the Face from Mask or Pressure

Masks cause less claustrophobia than the sensation of PAP therapy, so if you go slowly with the mask-fitting procedure, the anxiety and fear should not convert to claustrophobia. With the mask on, it should be clear that you can still breathe in and out, without the pressurized air, and you could make a case for easier breathing through a PAP mask than using a snorkeling system. Regardless, masks are designed for easy and rapid removal if you feel the need to do so.

Embarrassment, Shame, and Guilt. These emotions can cause big adaptation problems. You may not wish to discuss them with the sleep tech that night, or you may not experience them until you try PAP therapy at home. One irony about embarrassment relates to patients' fears of a negative impact on their sex lives, whereas PAP therapy has the distinct potential to add to your sex life by increasing your energy level and sex drive (libido). Cases have even described reversal of erectile dysfunction with PAP therapy. Given that more than 75 percent of patients at our sleep center report an unsatisfying decrease in their sex drive or sexual pleasure, PAP therapy could turn into a great motivator, given the possibility of it renewing one's romantic interests.

In the long run, love just might conquer all, but in the short run, a person with embarrassment or related feelings needs to address these issues, usually with those sharing the bed or bedroom. Occasionally we refer patients to marital therapy or couples counseling to resolve the impasse. Although these emotions are strong and very prevalent, scant research can be found in the scientific literature about this problem, which we imagine to be the greatest silent barrier to PAP therapy.

Imagery to the Rescue

All these emotions may reemerge when you start PAP therapy testing. We call this test a titration to determine pressurized airflow levels to produce normal breathing. The air sensation is difficult to describe, but some report it as similar to sticking your head out the window of a fast-moving car while trying to breathe. It is an unsettling feeling at first, primarily because breathing is the single most important physiological function over which you feel control. Anything that disrupts this control feeling, regardless of its illusory nature, causes alarm, because a threat is perceived. Most people settle down quickly to the sensation of air coming *in*, because you are also breathing *in*. Soon breathing in feels quite invigorating and may even create the feeling of breathing easier *in* with PAP therapy than without the device.

The biggest problem is breathing out against air coming in. The actual amount of pressurized airflow and the intensity of the pressure are very small and should not feel like a big deal. But anxiety and fear arrive on the scene and make pressurized airflow feel like a big deal. It is strange to breathe out against any amount of air coming in, and this strangeness produces a somatizing response in which susceptible individuals do not adapt well but instead focus attention on these strange feelings. The feelings intensify because an anxious mind deceives itself into thinking that the sensations are stronger than they really are.

When you feel feelings this way, it produces confusion, because you won't believe that the feelings can come and go. Your emotional response was probably triggered by your initial discomfort with the PAP mask, which then raised anxiety, which then increased tension in your airway, which then worsened pressure discomfort, which finally raised more anxiety, and so on.

To combat this problem, we teach PAP therapy users to distract themselves from the sensation of breathing out against pressurized airflow. By focusing elsewhere, the anxiety cycle is broken. The individual no longer notices the sensation as first experienced. Soon the sensation transforms into a feeling no different from normal breathing. We foster this change through imagery. Individuals are taught imagery exercises during a desensitization. If their skills are accessible, they image pleasant scenes for a minute to ten minutes while awake, breathing in and out with PAP therapy. Invariably they report a change in the way they perceive the sensation of breathing out against the airflow. Then we purposely have the patient stop imagery and notice the unpleasant feelings return, then restart the imagery to make unpleasant feelings subside. Eventually, these feelings completely disappear or at least no longer cause a problem.

This sequence builds confidence in patients, because they clearly see and feel their own reactions causing part or all of the uncomfortable sensations. They modify their reactions with imagery, giving them a real sense of control. If they have trouble with the exercise, they practice imagery prior to the test night, and then on the night of the test, we prepare them for frequent use of imagery. We also emphasize imagery exercises when using the mask in the first two to four weeks at home; the instructions for pleasant imagery practice in part three of the book suffice. Imagery work rapidly proves to the patient the psychophysiological nature of the anxiety due to breathing out against PAP therapy; and it shows how to dissolve the anxiety through pleasant imagery.

PAP-NAP on It

At some centers, you go through these desensitization procedures during the daytime and have the chance to nap with the mask strapped on and PAP therapy turned on (PAP-NAP). The purpose of the PAP-NAP is to give you an indication of your future experience in the lab. We feel that this procedure is critically important for heart patients and trauma patients, who seem to develop the most anxieties and fears about the entire breathing mask treatment.

For heart patients, we use this procedure because their SDB usually shows severe sleep apnea, and many of them suffer oxygen deficits in the severe, life-threatening range. We expect them to try the breathing mask halfway through the night—that is, in the split-night protocol. However, most heart patients are seasoned citizens; they have a lot of anxiety and fear about the mask. Using the short daytime PAP-NAP a few days before the split-night protocol gives them the chance to try PAP therapy for an hour or two and know what to expect.

For trauma patients, we start with the full-night diagnostic study; then, if anxiety is running high, we move to the PAP-NAP during the day. Only if the nap study was a successful experience for the patient would we schedule a full-night pressure titration. Otherwise we use other desensitization procedures or other treatments.

Airway Dynamics

When you breathe, special PAP mechanics must address the "switch" between air going in and air going out. CPAP manages this cycling by delivering a single, fixed-pressure level, measured in a unit called "centimeters of water," which stays the same. Pressure for most patients averages between 6 and 18 cms of H_2O, but some go lower and some go higher. If you use CPAP, you get only one pressure all night long. But logic suggests that many things in the human airway, including sleep position, stage of

---

SNOOZE FLASH
New PAP Pressure Delivery Systems

The ultimate key to your success with PAP therapy is finding the right *pressure delivery system* and the *right pressure settings*, both of which prove critical to splinting your airway in a stable position to remove any tendency toward collapsibility. When you think of the collapsible tube analogy, it sounds straightforward to picture greater air pressure going in, resulting in more stability of the airway. However, recent research on the dynamic and complex nature of airway physiology makes it clear that more advanced forms of PAP therapy are needed not only by cardiac patients or trauma survivors, but by many insomnia and other complex patients, too. CPAP as invented some thirty years ago was and still is a remarkable device that helps millions of people, but the newer pressure delivery systems have much to offer beyond simple CPAP.

Remember, you have to breathe in *and* out.

What we are now learning is that systems that ease the process of breathing out against PAP therapy coming *in* substantially increase your chances of using a device every night, all night. Moreover, it's now clear that the pressure needed to keep the airway open on expiration can be much lower than the pressure needed to keep it splinted on inspiration.

sleep, and variations in human anatomy require pressure to adapt at night.

Technological developments in this area have taken off and include devices that do some of the following:

- autoadjust pressure based on precise respiratory monitoring during sleep; the machine automatically changes in seconds to accommodate the need for lower or higher pressure;
    generally known as Automatic Positive Airway Pressure (APAP);
- exhalation relief in which the pressure automatically drops to a slightly lower level for a patient who cannot overcome discomfort in breathing out against air pressure coming in;
    trademarked as CFLEX devices or other brand names;
- two-level PAP therapy in which one pressure is set for inspiration and a second, lower pressure is set for expiration;
    generally known as Bilevel devices;
- volume-regulating machines, particularly helpful in central apnea;
    generally known as adapto-servo-ventilation (ASV).

Bilevel has been around for years, but this system is now increasingly used and is the subject of technological innovations as well. If you have any difficulty with CPAP, you might quickly turn things around by moving to one of these variations in pressure delivery.

Extras

We wish that mask and pressure issues were all you needed to figure out, but other factors radically influence your tolerance of PAP therapy, wearing the mask all night, and your overall response to treatment.

- *Ramps.* Hit a ramp button on your machine to start the pressure lower at bedtime. Gradually, over a few minutes or longer, pressure ramps to the proper settings, but presumably you fell asleep before it reached the final level, which may have initially bothered you. Ramps can be overused, and they may prevent you from adapting to the PAP pressures you need for a good treatment response. The most critical use of ramping occurs in the middle of the night when you awaken and feel uncomfortable with the pressure. The ramp delivers lower pressure while you return to sleep.

- *Humidifiers and Chinstraps.* Drying effects of pressurized air on the insides of your mouth or nose must be reduced. We recommend heated humidifiers with the PAP device. Drying sensations also are caused by mouth breathing, which is sufficiently irritating to wake you up. If nasal breathing is compromised, your body compensates by opening the mouth, which does not improve airflow enough to fix anything, but it does dry out your mouth. The harm caused by mouth breathing cannot be overestimated: if you require high pressures to overcome obstruction and resistance, and these pressures seem overpowering while asleep, you will open your mouth to release air pressure or draw in more air. Neither produces anything positive, as the loss of air pressure means that SDB is no longer treated. A chinstrap resolves mouth breathing, but it's another device to wear around your head, usually under the breathing mask to support the chin—not tightly—but enough to discourage mouth opening. Respironics Premium chinstrap is the best one we've used, because it creates the correct leverage to pull the chin up, not back.

- *Full Face Mask.* These masks fit over the nose and the mouth. They look monstrous; but remarkably, people with claustrophobia or mouth breathing find them comforting. They feel more confident in acquiring air through the nasal or oral airway. However, they are difficult to fit and may cause facial discomfort and pain. I rarely recommend full face masks except for those individuals who are obvious chronic mouth breathers *during the daytime*. Although these masks often leak air around edges, the full face may be the only solution for mouth breathers, whom we advise early in the course of treatment to see an ear, nose, and throat (ENT) physician.

Drying Things Up and Out

One of the maddening things about sorting out dry mouth problems is whether they are caused by mouth breathing or humidification. Generally, you detect a warmer feeling with dryness associated with a heated humidifier, whereas mouth breathing just produces dryness. With a humidifier, you also notice more areas of dryness in the nose or the back of the throat, whereas mouth breathing usually dries out the mouth.

The moisture from the humidifier can overcome dryness caused by pressurized air. For some people, no heating is required; rather, a passive system is used in which pressurized air runs through cold water to pick up sufficient moisture. Most patients find that heated humidifiers work best, but the technology for humidifiers is not advanced yet. They can be set too

PAP Therapy Checklist

During your first few weeks of PAP therapy, review this checklist every morning to track problems and progress.

PAP Therapy Follow-up Form

	None	Mild	Moderate	Severe
Mask Checklist				
1. Any pain	☐	☐	☐	☐
2. Any discomfort	☐	☐	☐	☐
3. Any air leakage	☐	☐	☐	☐
Air Pressure Checklist				
4. Any discomfort	☐	☐	☐	☐
5. Difficulty breathing out against the pressure	☐	☐	☐	☐

6. Your ability to adjust to the pressure (circle one)

   Very poor   Poor   Undecided   Good   Very good

Side Effects Checklist	None	Mild	Moderate	Severe
7. Sores or skin irritations from the mask	☐	☐	☐	☐
8. Air swallowing or bloating	☐	☐	☐	☐
9. Worsening of allergies, congestion, or sinus problems	☐	☐	☐	☐
10. Claustrophobia	☐	☐	☐	☐
11. Embarrassment	☐	☐	☐	☐

Impact Checklist

12. Hours slept _____

13. Hours of CPAP use _____

14. Sleep quality: (circle one)

    Very poor   Poor   Adequate   Fair   Good   Very good

15. How much benefit are you gaining from PAP therapy so far?

    None   Little   Moderate   Excellent   Outstanding

16. Level of motivation to continue: (circle one)

    Low Motivation   0   1   2   3   4   High Motivation

low and cause drying by lack of a moisturizing effect, or set too high and cause drying by heating up the nasal and oral airway. Frequently, humidifier settings must be changed every night to accommodate climate changes, although new devices adjust to the ambient humidity.

Most people need to go through periods of trial and error to sort out these effects, and most sleep physicians and sleep techs are capable in this realm and can help you tease apart the problems and find precise solutions.

SLEEP ON IT
The Morning After

QUESTION: The big question the morning after your first night of PAP therapy is whether you can tell any differences in how you slept. You might think this change would be easy to spot, but guess again. What we've noticed is that a fair number of people—easily 25 percent or greater—cannot see any difference until about five that afternoon—that is, the afternoon after waking up from the test.

Because sensors and wires are so intrusive and annoying, many people do not notice that sleep was more refreshing or deeper. Only later that afternoon do they notice more zip, less sleepiness and fatigue, and sometimes greater mental sharpness. All after just one night.

Unfortunately, many people do not have a consistent night of good sleep in the lab with their first use of PAP therapy, but the technician usually has gathered sufficient data for the doctor to write a prescription to start therapy at home. Less commonly, the test goes so poorly that the patient must return for another titration study to test pressures before starting at home. After your first night of PAP therapy and after successive nights at home, can you motivate yourself to use the CPAP checklist every morning to help fine-tune your adaptation by targeting specific barriers?

COMMENT: Please notice how the form converges around three major areas:

1. discomfort or pain and anxiety or fear with mask fitting;
2. discomfort or pain and anxiety or fear with pressurized airflow;
3. sense of embarrassment versus progress and motivation to continue.

─────── PEARL ───────
Curiosity, Flexibility, and a
Medication Reprieve

The secret to success with PAP is maintaining a high curiosity level about the whole experience, especially for the first few days and weeks. If any question arises, don't let it slide. Monitor the issue for no more than three days, and often for just one day; then phone your home care company (the place where you got the PAP device from and described in the next chapter) or your sleep center for advice. The longer you leave things unsettled, the more you'll develop frustrations and self-defeating learned behaviors, which lead you to resent if not despise the breathing mask treatment.

By maintaining a high level of curiosity, you spot specific obstacles. It may be as simple as tightening your chinstrap, turning up the humidifier half a notch, or repositioning your mask in front of a mirror. Never underestimate the minutiae, because the details of using PAP therapy almost always need attention to achieve *Sound Sleep*. And once you achieve sound sleep, the minutiae will be well worth it, because the little things take less than two minutes per day.

A special note here if you suffer from air swallowing from PAP therapy that causes you bloated feelings in the morning. This may be due to leg jerks, so please note the information in chapter 29, on page 291, to resolve this problem.

Another consideration is your flexibility. The last thing you want is to drive yourself nuts trying out PAP therapy. Few people learn to use the device by barreling ahead, pushing themselves to the limit. Instead, they make their sleep worse, grow to hate CPAP, and then swear they'll never try it or anything else again in their efforts to overcome SDB. Curiosity and flexibility are needed to maintain your interest and build a schedule that works to win the war, because you should expect to lose several battles or at least a few skirmishes along the way in trying to adapt to PAP therapy.

For a very important segment of users, you may be the type who would actually be served well by staying on or perhaps starting a sedating type of medication until you have fully adapted to PAP therapy. In fact, recent research suggests that some SDB patients suffer from a pernicious arousal pattern known as "cyclic alternating pattern" or CAP, which often retards their progress in using PAP therapy. Among the latest research studies, some of these patients responded much more favorably and consistently using a sedative or sedating antide-pressants along with PAP therapy. Do not view these findings as in conflict with earlier points about sleep medication. Some individuals really do respond better to drugs than to various psychological treatments. Therefore, this combination approach may be best for some PAP users.

Last, once you taste *Sound Sleep*, it is imperative to sense whether you are gaining more delta sleep (more restorative slumber) or more REM sleep (more dream awareness). Fine-tuning pressures in the sleep lab will aid this process. Or, you can clarify things by using your SOLO skills to note how rested you feel and how much you have been dreaming. Strangely, you can sometimes sleep so deeply with PAP therapy, you experience "sleep inertia" soon after awakening in the morning. Sleep iner-tia is different from refreshing sleep; it just means you take longer to get started in the morning, but your energy is strong once you get moving. Last, use the SDB-28 weekly to monitor changes in symptoms and related progress.

28

Welcome to Your Home Health Company

Prescriptions

To obtain a PAP device and all related equipment requires a prescription written by a doctor, who may be a sleep physician or your primary-care physician. Once written, it goes to a home health company that sells durable medical equipment (DME), and they also supply things such as wheelchairs, crutches, and oxygen tanks. Usually the DME company and your insurance carrier require additional documentation of your sleep study results to move forward.

To get your breathing mask, lots of steps are needed, in the following sequence:

- The sleep tech completes the PAP titration sleep study.
- The sleep tech manually scores the sleep study.
- The sleep physician reads and reviews the sleep study and prepares the final report.
- The sleep physician usually discusses the results with the patient to determine interest and motivation to use PAP therapy, and then writes a prescription.
- At the sleep center, the prescription goes to a patient care coordinator or a clerk, who completes more paperwork.
- The prescription and the sleep study results are sent to the DME company.

- The DME company contacts the insurance carrier to seek approval.
- The insurance carrier contacts the DME (from one to thirty days later) to authorize equipment.
- The DME contacts the sleep center or the patient about the insurance approval.
- The DME or the sleep center arranges for the patient to go to the DME office to pick up equipment and to learn instructions on use.

There are several flaws in this system, the most obvious the bureaucratic quagmire that prevents you from striking while the iron is hot. If you had a positive PAP therapy response, it is to your advantage to start the next night. Some programs send out loaner machines with patients to tide them over, while some sleep centers own their own DME companies and initiate PAP therapy quickly. Many operations, though, suffer from intolerable waits. Imagine for a moment a doctor diagnosing you with diabetes, but you have to wait weeks to get your insulin and related supplies. If you got sick and landed in the hospital, do you know how many lawyers would be licking their chops to take your case? But if you think the wait is bad, it pales in comparison to the most serious flaws in the system.

DME Companies

In sleep medicine, we have concerns about DME companies and the support they may or may not provide to our sleep patients. These issues are complex and controversial because they involve Medicare policymakers along with other insurance carriers. Currently, there is not a consistently satisfying system in place to efficiently use the sleep medicine community to help SDB patients adapt to their PAP therapy devices. Instead, insurance carriers, including Medicare, have set up a policy that technically and financially grants too much responsibility to the DME companies and their staff to aid patients' efforts. This odd arrangement originally derived from the premise that breathing equipment seems similar to other medical equipment, such as wheelchairs, crutches, and oxygen concentrators. That is, the patient rents, buys, or leases equipment and uses it for a time. The paradox is that patients learn to use crutches in a matter of minutes or wheelchairs in hours; whereas, PAP therapy adaptation and regular use requires one to three months of dedicated effort. Such attempts are exasperating for complex patients with SDB, who also suffer from insomnia or depression or posttraumatic stress disorder. Unlike using a pair of crutches, the adaptation for such patients requires constant fiddling with the equipment, repeated adjustments to device settings, and retitrations in the sleep lab during the first few months of use.

The field of sleep medicine continues to ask: who are the best providers to help sleep patients learn to use PAP therapy? But this question is not the one asked by insurance companies who cover much of the costs of this equipment. Remarkably, the system was created so that DME companies are not only reimbursed for equipment, but they also receive an allotment built into their reimbursements to cover their costs to teach patients how to use PAP therapy. Yet, it is not clear how much the average DME company specializes in PAP therapy equipment and how well their staff are trained to provide these services. I've never heard of any DME company training its staff to teach PTSD patients how to use PAP therapy. In some states, the law requires a respiratory therapist at the DME company to teach the SDB patient, but this specialized therapist may have never worked in a sleep center and therefore may have less skill than a sleep tech.

Sleep techs, under the supervision of sleep physicians or other healthcare providers, are the logical choice to help SDB patients, but insurance companies have not established the means to reimburse for sleep tech services. They pay for physicians, physician assistants, nurse practitioners and nurses to interact with sleep patients, but these professionals are costly to engage for this type of service. Regardless, sleep techs, in my experience, are usually more skilled than any of these providers in teaching patients how to use PAP therapy. And, why not, all night long they fit and test literally thousands of patients in a perfect hands-on environment. How could they not be the most skilled professionals for such efforts? To repeat, though, a sleep tech's work in a sleep lab is only counted toward billing and reimbursement when they work to conduct sleep tests, not to assist patients during daytime clinics.

In a recent development, Medicare has started looking into quality issues to evaluate services of DME companies providing PAP therapy equipment. I am concerned they are not looking for ways to maximize the contributions of sleep techs. It is ironic and discouraging that the individuals with the most experience and skill as well as the lowest salaries in the sleep medical field are essentially shut out from financial process. Sleep techs have a great deal to offer, but currently sleep centers can only offer their services free of charge.

Locally Owned and Operated

In time, it would be invaluable if DME companies and sleep medical facilities could find ways to more closely collaborate to improve patient care. Unfortunately or not, the actions of those DMEs that provide limited or weak services seem to have spurred many sleep medical centers and labs to open their own DME branches to gain control of the process. This trend appears to be a wave of the future, so if you discover a sleep facility that handles DME, you may find they offer greater expertise on sleep equipment and related services.

In the meantime, you are most likely to find yourself working with a locally owned or franchised DME company in your city. In Albuquerque, we consistently see that locally owned home health equipment companies make the most concerted efforts to improve the skills of their respiratory therapists. In contrast, nationally franchised companies that set up shops all over the country have a weaker track record in our city and around our state; these franchises demonstrate inconsistent abilities and often show a lot of ignorance about the latest advances in PAP therapy devices and in mask technology. They also seem to make their patients wait longer for equipment and services. Because they are a franchise, they contract with insurance companies by offering better prices, but lower price might yield lower quality of care. If you scout out locally owned companies in your area, you might find more suitable care.

SNOOZE FLASH

Coverage of PAP Therapy for UARS

Despite all the DME and insurance snafus, none is more disquieting than not being able to get your equipment at all or not being able to get the right equipment. A classic example would be the upper airway resistance patient, who is dealing with his insurance carrier's medical director, who might be a cardiologist, who has never heard of upper airway resistance. The doctor would only know about counting up apneas and hypopneas in the Respiratory Disturbance Index. If apneas and hypopneas are all that are counted, the UARS events would be left out of the equation, giving a false impression of SDB severity. And Medicare and some insurance companies will not pay for patients to use PAP therapy if they suffer only from UARS.

Acquiring Standard and Advanced PAP Devices

In a UARS situation, the only way you obtain a PAP device in some cities is through your sleep physician going to bat for you, and usually the sleep doctor will have to push pretty hard. For some, you will need to pay for the device yourself. In Albuquerque, we have discussed the issue of upper airway resistance and clarified our protocols with all the medical directors. They found the material informative, and most accepted the terminology and the PAP prescription. Yet some patients waited months to get a PAP device. A similar issue involves asking your insurance carrier to give coverage on an advanced technological device such as APAP or Bilevel. We now write APAP or Bilevel prescriptions routinely for insomniacs, and most but not all the insurance carriers accept our prescriptions without delay.

You should realize that acceptance does not equate to costs. Some DME companies use this opportunity to charge more money, because these devices are more expensive for them to buy and inventory. In time, more advanced devices will probably become less expensive, because newer, still more advanced devices will take their place.

Crucial to your efforts, if you have trouble adjusting to standard, fixed CPAP, you absolutely want to find a way to try another pressure delivery system. Often arrangements can be worked out to rent a different device for one month, such as APAP or Bilevel, before committing to buying a more expensive machine. It is truly worth its weight in gold to use one of these devices if it helps you sleep all night long.

Follow-up, Follow-up, Follow-up

To maximize your chances of using PAP therapy, you must have a clear-cut follow-up plan in place with your sleep center, sleep lab, or other medical clinic. If you are lucky, and your DME supplier has an experienced respiratory therapist who really knows the ins and outs of PAP therapy equipment, then you would be in the minority but fortunate nonetheless. For some people, on-site evaluations and adjustments are critical, while for others, it's a matter of brief phone calls or e-mails.

Follow-up is essential in the first days, weeks, or month, because these intervals reflect the period when patients often make decisions to stop using PAP therapy, undoubtedly because they are not getting a good response, or worse, because it aggravated their sleep problems. Solving PAP therapy problems requires time, energy, money, and a commitment to achieve a goal of using your therapy every night for the whole night.

Although there are countless issues that may need to be addressed, use your daily PAP Therapy Checklist in conjunction with the following questions to monitor things closely in the first few days, weeks, or month:

- Does your PAP pressure setting seem too high or too low?
- Do you notice air leakage from any other location on the mask, besides the normal air leak vent that permits removal of carbon dioxide?
- Is the mask coming off at night without your awareness?
- Is the mask continuing to cause discomfort or pain?
- Are you wearing the mask all night but not feeling like your sleep quality is any better?
- Are you experiencing any signs of mouth breathing?
- Are you swallowing air and having a distended stomach in the morning?
- Are your legs jerking at night?
- Is your frustration with the experience reaching a breaking point?

You need time to adjust, but these elements could also be barriers that prevent you from adjusting. When you notice problems based on the questions above, don't wait to take action. These factors are important indicators that the adaptation may *not* be going well and that you need advice sooner, not later.

Again, a reminder to use the SDB-28 to monitor changes in symptoms to help you recognize whether you are achieving substantial benefits.

Take Another Breather

Many people cannot adjust to PAP devices right away or even in a few months. During the time of their difficulties, they usually build up a new set of learned behaviors along with negative feelings about the device. Once these habits and emotions become entrenched, it is difficult to succeed even if you start on a more advanced device, because your aggravation about the whole thing may be more intense than you realize, and your sleep may worsen.

What's the answer?

Take a break from PAP devices. Even if you intend to switch to a new device, you need to clarify in your own mind and body just how much damage has been done by your first experience with PAP therapy. If you feel highly motivated to move on to the next device and don't sense too much frustration or aggravation with fixed CPAP, by all means move ahead. But if you feel like you worked hard, yet things got worse, then you are a setup for having no luck with the next device.

The break might last a week, a month, or more. The short version of the break means giving yourself a breather, focusing on nasal strips, a chinstrap, and the position you sleep in. More importantly, it means working through the unpleasant emotions you have built up about your first experience so you can become ready, willing, and able to move on. The longer version of the break, which may be suitable for many problematic sleepers, is to explore a completely different pathway to treat SDB—one into which many find they can really sink their teeth.

Oral Appliance Therapy

Oral appliance therapy (OAT) is truly a godsend for some people, because you wear a piece of plastic fit to your teeth to hold your jaw in a thrusted position to enhance breathing during sleep. Remarkably, it is a dental device for a medical condition, and most insurance companies, but not all, cover it under durable medical equipment; and many insurance companies pay at least 50 percent of the costs.

What's exciting about OAT is that if it works well, you have almost no awareness of using it until removed in the morning, after which you feel soreness in the back of your jaw, lasting a few minutes up to a few hours. This soreness is the key to whether you can use such a device, because the impact on your temporomandibular joint (TMJ) ultimately determines OAT tolerance.

Most OAT devices move the lower jaw (mandible) forward, stabilize it in a thrusted position, and thereby expand the airway in the back of your throat. But if you suffer from TMJ problems, as many insomnia or mental health patients do, OAT may be the devil in disguise. So listen carefully before you consider OAT.

When an OAT device is fitted improperly or by a dentist with limited experience treating TMJ dysfunction, the device won't work well, and it injures or worsens TMJ, setting you back months or years. TMJ dysfunction does not automatically preclude OAT, but ideally you will work with a dentist who treats TMJ dysfunction and has made oral appliances for such patients. Pursuing this level of expertise is essential to ensure the best assessment of your tolerance to OAT (unless you do not have TMJ problems). Then, if you are fitted for one, you will be in the best hands for receiving follow-up care. Regrettably, this combined level of expertise may be a rare thing to find in your community, but forewarned is forearmed.

OAT Specifications

The best dental devices are made with standard dental impression molds of upper and lower teeth. There also are boil-and-bite types. This device is softened in hot water; then, while still malleable, it is placed in your mouth for an instant fit. After you remove it from your mouth, it hardens and stays in that shape. These boil-and-bite devices are far less expensive than lab-built types, but they are less effective in comfort and treatment impact on SDB. I recommend lab-built Silencer, EMA, Klearway, and TAPS as advanced, reliable, and effective devices. I know of their effectiveness in my patients or in my colleagues' patients, especially those in the field of dental sleep medicine. There are many more devices that undoubtedly have proven capabilities.

OAT is best suited for people with less severe SDB. They may be ideal for UARS patients, some of whom should start with dental devices instead of PAP therapy. They work for patients who have apneas and hypopneas, but the greater the SDB severity, then usually the lesser the impact. OAT success is anatomy- and physiology-dependent. Obese patients with thick necks might suffer only from UARS, but the pressure from adipose tissues in the neck or airway diminishes the impact of OAT. A thorough exam by a dentist who regularly offers OAT is advised to make the most accurate determination on using such devices. Even if your personal dentist is great, you may be better off with a dentist who has fitted OAT for twenty-five to fifty other patients.

The most frequent side effect is alteration in your bite in the morning, which can produce long-term changes. In the morning, you learn not to eat toast or chewy or crunchy things, because your teeth don't line up properly, causing you to bite your lips or your cheeks. Over time this problem worsens into an open bite in which affected teeth, usually upper and lower molars, no longer meet and touch when you close your mouth. Instead, they remain apart even when you bite down.

After you remove the dental device in the morning, you can bite down on a small piece of hard but malleable plastic between your upper front teeth and lower front teeth, which then has the effect of pushing the lower jaw back into its usual position. The plastic is about 1 to 2 cm wide and about 2 to 3 cm long; the piece rests behind (posterior to) the upper front teeth and in front (anterior to) the lower front teeth. Used for a few minutes or for up to fifteen minutes after removing the dental device diminishes bite problems.

Some people alternate devices, using PAP therapy for a few weeks followed by OAT for a few weeks or on other schedules. This pathway limits dental occlusion problems, and it facilitates adaptation by allowing you to take a break from each device until you gain comfort with one or both systems. The critical decision on OAT comes down to what to try first. We persuade most patients to try PAP first, but a case can be made to bypass it and go directly to OAT. Here's a list of factors that may lean you toward OAT first:

- Your perceptions of CPAP make you believe you would never be able to use a PAP device, for whatever reason or reasons.
- Your Respiratory Disturbance Index is less than thirty events per hour, and most of the events are UARS, with few hypopneas or apneas.
- Your oxygen level does not drop below 90 percent, or if it does go into the high 80 percent range, these desaturations are infrequent.
- You have good dentition, no or minimal TMJ problems, and very little if any removable prosthetic teeth, such as dentures.
- You travel frequently or to places without electricity.

Milder SDB conditions might do better with OAT. If your instincts move you toward this method, be sure to discuss this possibility with your sleep physician, who usually must write a referral or a prescription to obtain OAT fitted by a dentist. Other devices also are on the market, such as tongue retaining devices (TRDs), and although less widely used than OAT, they may work for certain individuals. More devices are being tested for SDB, and these devices use other mechanical systems unrelated to or combined with PAP therapy systems.

SLEEP ON IT
Helpful Hints

QUESTION: These helpful hints assume you have started using a PAP device or are just about to start, so please refer back to the items discussed here, if applicable. Many people discover factors affecting their use of the device after they start using it. That's no surprise, but for some people it may be profitable to examine concerns about your machine before you obtain, rent, or buy it. The good news is that many DME companies rent or lease the equipment to you before you buy it. Thus you have more opportunities to discover factors to change. If you have started with a machine, does anything come to mind already that you would like to change?

COMMENT: With every step you take, keep in mind a key point about sleep quantity. Recall how we discussed that a sleeper doesn't really know the hours of sleep needed each night until he or she learns to sleep soundly through the night. PAP therapy may confuse you because you could start sleeping longer if your body seeks to catch up on old sleep debt. With breathing stabilized, you could have the unsettling but pleasurable experience of revisiting your youth, finding yourself one morning awakening after sleeping nine, ten, eleven, or twelve hours. Just the opposite can occur: you sleep less because your sleep quality is so much better. You no longer need as much sleep, yet your energy level is as high as or higher than it has ever been.

Don't worry about or be alarmed by changes in your sleep quantity at this point because, as always, enhancing sleep quality is the secret to *Sound Sleep*. Instead, use your new appreciation for the fuller depth of sleep quality to make fine-tuning adjustments to your PAP therapy.

——— PEARL ———

Know Your PAP Device Like the Front of Your Face

You are going to become intimate with your PAP device, so you need to think in terms of simple things that could enhance or detract from your experience. Let's run down key elements:

- *Cleaning.* Clean the tubes and mask after each use. You can use 1:10 vinegar and water or something stronger, such as an antibacterial soap. Some tubes and masks are more difficult to clean and take more time, but it is more comforting to crawl into bed and feel a clean mask on your face and air coming through clean tubes.
- *Filters.* Most people forget to change them as recommended at least once per month. Dust certainly settles on top of the device as it sits by your bed, so it is a maintenance necessity to have the filter working properly in the PAP device.

- *Noise.* When delivering the pressurized airflow into the tube, air compressors emit far less sound than the machines built just a few years back. If the sound or the pitch is still too bothersome, use earplugs with the PAP device. Earplugs rated for thirty-one decibels or greater are needed, and they should have a porous look to their surface, as this patterning decreases irritation to the ear canal. Custom-fitted earplugs are best but more expensive.

- *Size/Weight.* I travel everywhere with my PAP device (Puritan Bennett Goodknight 425 Bilevel) except on camping trips, when I'll use my oral appliance, the Silencer. Puritan Bennett devices are the most compact and lightest and smaller than all other machines. Regardless, all machines can be packed in tote bags and carried on an airplane, because it is prudent not to stow them with luggage.

- *Positioning.* If you place your PAP device to the side of the bed, which may be the only convenient spot, you may discover some hindrance in turning to one side or another. Or you may discover that you roll onto the tubing. The ideal way to position the device is at the head of the bed. I converted a computer bookshelf into a modified headboard. The PAP device and the humidifier sit on the shelf, which is about six to eight inches below the top of the mattress. However, the PAP device also sits on a couple of thick books to raise it above the humidifier. This height difference aids the way in which the humidifier operates, and by having all the equipment at the head of my bed, I can easily keep the tubes out of my way. I also can reach my machine in case I need to fiddle with the humidifier during the night or use the ramp button.

- *Data Download.* The Puritan Bennett Goodknight 420E APAP device is a good system, which records nightly usage figures as well as measuring apneas, hypopneas, and UARS events. It also detects air leakage and mouth breathing. However, these data are not perfected yet, so you cannot clarify all issues at home. You will see patterns of pressure too high or too low or that you are mouth breathing, so your doctor can adjust the machine some-what before recommending another night in the sleep lab.

Many of these factors can throw you for a loop when you try to use a PAP device, but once you approach these elements in an organized manner, you find the experience is not as overwhelming as it sounds. If you obtain real benefits from your device, your motivation skyrockets to take care of the equipment. Once it all comes together, you spend as little as two to no more than ten minutes per day fiddling with your PAP therapy equipment.

The last and sometimes most important pearl to remember is to find the proper dose of PAP therapy and never overdose yourself in the early going. One patient was so nervous, she only used PAP therapy on weekends for three months before gaining confidence to use it during the week. And one patient with claustrophobia was capable only of putting on the mask and turning on the pressure while sitting up in bed and reading for an hour. Then she removed it and went to sleep. After several weeks, her anxieties decreased, and she was willing to progress.

Slow and steady is universally the best approach to initiating and adapting to PAP therapy for reluctant users. For those without any barriers, rapid use brings rapid results that maximize their motivation within days of starting.

29

Moving On Up

Getting a Leg Up

Restless legs syndrome (RLS) and periodic limb movement disorder (PLMD) are the other two common physical sleep disorders, affecting tens of millions of people. Both conditions lead to movement of the legs. Neither condition has a full explanation for why it occurs. Yet both conditions are adequately treated with low doses of specialized medication.

RLS is the condition in which:

- While lying or sitting, uncomfortable or difficult-to-describe sensations occur in the back of the calves (or in other spots on the leg or arms), so unpleasant you must move your body.
- Movement of the legs, arms, or body eliminates the feeling.
- The sensation returns when you stop moving.
- The sensation intensifies during the evening or at bedtime.
- The feeling prevents sleep or makes it difficult to sleep.

RLS is a waking condition; it occurs prior to sleep, whereas PLMD is a sleeping condition in which:

- Legs jerk or twitch rhythmically (periodically) during the night.
- The leg jerk may be small and barely noticeable, occurring in the ankle or involving dramatic motions in the whole body.
- Each movement lasts a few seconds or less.

- The movements occur in repeating cycles, say, once every thirty seconds—with cycles usually ranging in the thirty- to ninety-second time frame.
- The movements may or may not provoke an arousal discernible in the EEG—that is, speeding up the brain waves.
- The impact of PLMD on sleep is controversial, but it produces enough disruption in some sleep-disordered breathing (SDB) patients to prevent CPAP use, and it may disrupt sleep in patients without SDB.

If you have RLS, there's a high chance you have PLMD during sleep. Those with PLMD have a 50 percent chance of also suffering from RLS.

Crazy Legs

Both conditions are quite real. At their worst, RLS drives a person into a state of mental instability, because it is so harrowing not to know what's causing it or how to stop it. RLS is easily missed because so few physicians are aware of it, although recent advertising has improved awareness. Patients think it a weird complaint and often endure it for years, compensating in various ways. The most disabling problem is staying up later and later, so total sleep declines.

Many with RLS use drugs or alcohol to sleep, which often compounds the problem. Many physicians have prescribed sedatives or antidepressants for these patients without ever hearing about the leg-movement part of the sleep complaint. Sedatives are fairly weak treatments for RLS in comparison to well-researched treatments. Antidepressants cause or aggravate RLS or PLMD symptoms in some patients.

Both RLS and PLMD lead to psychiatric symptoms such as anxiety or depression, which may be due to lack of sleep or the impact of the strange feelings. The overall psychological impairment, most commonly in terms of anxiety or depression, has been described as equal to other patients with depression or diabetes.

Controversy surrounds both conditions. RLS has been satirized by misinformed talk-radio hosts, and serious questions have arisen in the sleep medicine community about the clinical import of PLMD.

SNOOZE FLASH

The Link between SDB and Leg Jerks

The great controversy about RLS and PLMD is their relationship to SDB. Many patients with RLS and PLMD also suffer from SDB, especially upper airway resistance events. In sleep studies in some of these patients, recent research shows that the movement occurred at the end of a UARS event. Remarkably, when these patients received PAP therapy, their leg jerks decreased as air pressure normalized breathing. Of further interest, research also has shown the opposite result, in which a PLMD patient with SDB was treated with a medication to eliminate leg jerks, which then stabilized sleep and eliminated SDB. Chart 5 on page 262 shows examples of how leg jerks appear on the sleep test and how they interact with SDB events.

Breathless Legs

These SDB findings indicate that some people's conditions mimic but are not true leg movement disorders. This conundrum requires patience to sort out at a sleep center. If we see PLMD in an SDB patient, we are reluctant to treat the legs until we've treated the breathing. But if the patient also complains of RLS, then the leg jerks are more suspicious. Then we could start medication before the first night of PAP therapy, so that when next tested in the lab, we determine whether the drug decreased leg jerks. Usually, if the patient reports that the drug decreased RLS, the sleep test confirms that the leg jerks decreased, too.

The most important consideration in SDB cases is whether RLS or PLMD interfere with PAP therapy. In those with clear-cut cases of restless legs or leg jerks, then the proper medication transforms their use of PAP therapy. You will be surprised to know which medication achieves these dramatic results, and you already know it is not sedatives.

Medications

Fortunately, a single drug from several choices treats either or both RLS or PLMD. In severe cases, a patient may use two medications or alternate drugs. The list of available drugs is growing longer with increasing research and interest in movement disorders. We'll focus on proven medications that actually eliminate RLS or PLMD feelings or movements.

Carbidopa/Levodopa or Sinemet is the granddaddy medication, having been used successfully for decades to treat RLS or PLMD. It works through dopamine (a neurotransmitter) pathways, and newer drugs for movement disorders work on these dopaminergic pathways as well. Sinemet or variations of it are taken thirty minutes before bedtime, and a repeat dose can be used a few hours later if awakened by leg jerks; or a long-acting version works for some and obviates use of the second dose. The problems with Sinemet are side effects, many of which are minor and often resolve in a week or two. Most notable is nausea or vomiting. But Sinemet also has serious side effects, the worst of which is worsening of RLS to earlier in the day. If the drug is not stopped, RLS occurs 24/7. This side effect can develop into an emergency, because the patient may become mentally unstable with round-the-clock RLS. This "augmentation" effect means that the drug cannot be used again. Other side effects include increased risk for depression or suicidal thinking and neurologic symptoms such as various movement disorders, including a greater risk for seizures if you currently suffer from seizures.

Newer dopaminergic agents include pramipexole (Mirapex) and ropinirole (Requip), which have excellent safety profiles. You must start with the lowest dose for about a week and assess impact on RLS, then increase over time. This pattern also reduces side effects. Requip is unique in that it is taken one hour to three hours before bedtime.

Sleeping Pills Not

It is fascinating to hear patients talk about how these dopaminergic drugs work. They all expect a sedative-like effect. Instead, the pills work as if you were uncovering a disguised emotion that was blocking the *Wave of Sleepiness*. In this case, the feeling of restless legs blocks your *Wave*. Once the drug eliminates RLS, the *Wave* laps upon the shore, and the patient falls asleep. Most patients are surprised by this sequence, even though they were told the drug is not a sedative. That's why the medication is taken before bedtime, not at bedtime.

A final drug to mention is oxycodone, which raises red flags in many people's minds, as it is a narcotic. But remember, treatment of RLS or PLMD usually responds to low doses of drugs. Oxycodone pills are prescribed in very low doses compared to that for someone with a broken ankle. The latter patient would receive a bottle of sixty pills in one week. In contrast, sixty pills would last an RLS patient a month to two months. A sleep physician would not prescribe more than this amount except for a rare individual who might require three or four pills per night. Since learning about the relationship between PLMD and UARS, I have not prescribed more than two oxycodone pills per night for any patient.

Abuse potential is very low, because the patient will not be able to persuade the sleep physician to prescribe more. Patients can always doctor-shop for more, but then signs of addiction or dependency show up. In my clinical experience, addiction or dependency problems are extremely rare in patients prescribed oxycodone for RLS or PLMD. Oxycodone is safe, but it can produce the troubling side effect of constipation. It also imparts some sedating feelings, especially in the first few days or weeks of use. More importantly, it eliminates RLS and PLMD, so drug-induced sleepiness is a small if not inconsequential part of the mechanism.

Numerous medications are in use for RLS or PLMD, but those discussed are the most established and effective. Sleep specialists keep current on medication research for movement disorders, because most centers see at least 10 percent of patients with these problems.

Medication is all that's needed when movement disorders are independent with no SDB. With the advent of pressure transducer technology for measuring breathing, we see many more cases of PLMD interrelated with SDB. Thus many patients use PAP therapy and RLS/PLMD drugs. And this combination of treatment is especially important to mention in light of an unusual side effect to PAP therapy known as air swallowing. It seems that many cases of air swallowing are caused by leg jerks, where the jerking motion causes the person to awaken and swallow air, which can cause painful bloating. By treating the leg jerks effectively, air swallowing is often eliminated.

Natural Therapies

Vitamin and mineral deficiencies are implicated in RLS or PLMD:

- iron storage, measured by ferritin levels;
- magnesium;
- folate;
- vitamin B_{12}.

This bloodwork may need to be tested, particularly if there is a history of anemia, which might signal iron or vitamin deficiencies. Magnesium tests are rarely low unless caused by other disease or drugs, yet of interest, magnesium supplements have improved RLS, and more so for PLMD in patients without low magnesium levels. No controlled studies have been conducted with this mineral supplement.

The most interesting area of recent research theorizes an iron-dopamine connection to RLS. One dramatic report showed RLS developing in patients with acute blood loss, which would have produced a low iron state. Then the movement symptoms were eliminated following blood transfusions that resupplied iron levels.

Ferritin is a marker of iron storage and has been used to indicate a low iron state in RLS patients. The most recent cutoff is 45 to 50 ng/ml (nanograms per milliliter), wherein a ferritin level near or below this number may indicate possible benefit for an RLS patient who wants to consider iron supplements. Remarkably, you do not need to have anemia to also have a low ferritin level.

Iron supplementation is not a trivial matter. Excessive iron accumulation in the body is dangerous, and iron supplements in your house can be dangerous to children or to anyone else who accidentally ingests it. It is essential to discuss supplemental iron with your sleep or primary physician; it is not something to try without gathering more information and lab work.

SLEEP ON IT
Walking It Off

QUESTION: Assessing the need for RLS or PLMD medication can range in complexity to a walk in the garden to one through a labyrinth. In addition to all the factors listed, the use of antidepressants often produces great confusion about leg movements. Do you take an antidepressant? If so, review this material closely if you suffer from RLS or PLMD.

COMMENT: On a sleep test, many patients using psychotropic medications demonstrate leg jerks (PLMD), particularly those patients using antidepressant medications. This information is not widely known in the mental health community, or if it is known, it is not viewed as a problem. Not all antidepressants cause leg jerks, but many, particularly the selective serotonin reuptake inhibitor (SSRI) medications, appear to induce leg jerks during sleep. We often see a great increase in leg jerk frequency on sleep tests, yet sometimes without the expected arousals. The questions for troubled sleepers are whether they should switch medication to one without this side effect, or whether the leg jerks have no impact on sleep. Perhaps the leg jerks were always there, and the antidepressant made them worse.

———— PEARL ————
Antidepressant Users Step Forward

These questions are not easy to sort through, but mental health patients who use antidepressants must address them in the following contexts:

- Is the antidepressant producing clear-cut improvements in depression?
- Is it worth changing medication to find one yielding clearer improvement?
- Is it feasible to stop medication completely to see the impact on leg jerks?
- Is it feasible to stop medication and use emotional processing skills as an alternative to antidepressant medication?
- If the medication is working well and should be maintained, would there be a value to adding another medication to treat the leg jerks?

Many mental health patients and other troubled sleepers with the combination of SDB and leg movements must sort out the impact of each disorder. This step may take months. In my first case with this level of complexity, it took two years to help the patient off of three medications while starting her on two new ones and at the same time help her with PAP therapy struggles. Finally she selected oral appliance therapy. The difficulties arose because her medications were clearly helping her depression but also making her sleep much worse, with high-frequency leg jerks. When her medication was changed, her depression often got worse, even though her leg jerks were decreasing in frequency and her sleep was getting better.

We clearly saw a large improvement in her sleep consolidation and a decrease in her leg jerks and arousals once she was stabilized on a combination of OAT, medications for psychiatric disorders, and a drug for RLS and PLMD.

For mental health patients, in particular, this process takes considerable time, frequent sleep testing in the lab, and several physician encounters, but the results are well worth it.

30

The Long and Winding Road

The Journey Begins

You have traveled a long way searching for *Sound Sleep* and the *Sound Mind* that follows. Regardless of your progress, the more important question is whether you see the light at the end of the tunnel. Many are in various stages of sleep-disordered breathing (SDB) treatment by now or have started medication for leg movement disorders. Some are still navigating their way through sleep center consultations, while still others might be waiting for first contact with a sleep center or a lab. Some poor sleepers need more time and reflection to sort out whether to move forward with an evaluation for physiological sleep disorders.

Wherever you are on the path, sometimes you must return to pertinent sections of the book to solidify and enhance your progress. Never hesitate to return to essential passages, particularly Little Big Steps, Pearls, and Snooze Flashes, which were written for repeat reading and review to help along this path—which in reality is the beginning of the journey, not the end.

Most problematic sleepers have learned to appreciate that getting the sleep you need is vital to your mood, well-being, and energy level, not to mention its impact on your heart and brain and your mental and physical health. Based on all you are hopefully experiencing, sleep is now as important to you as exercise, diet, and stress reduction programs, because maximizing *Sound Sleep* provides the energy, concentration, and inner resolve to foster the attitudes and skills to exercise frequently, eat right, and cope with emotions more usefully.

A pot of gold really is waiting at the end of your sleep rainbow, but now you know that a lifelong commitment is needed to gain *Sound Sleep* and take advantage of the wondrous impact it has on the rest of your life.

SNOOZE FLASH

A Surgeon's Knife Cuts Both Ways

A fair proportion of problematic sleepers discover that PAP therapy and OAT still seem too far beyond their grasp. Given the potential awkwardness of these devices, it is no surprise that some troubled sleepers just cannot use them. Many want surgery, which is not unreasonable on a theoretical level but often turns out to be highly impractical on the local level.

Unless surgeons have worked in the field of sleep medicine, they are prone to making blanket statements about how such-and-such a procedure proves useful for SDB. Yet, data are often lacking to support their claims. Take the procedure known as UPPP or U-TripleP (uvulopalatopharyngoplasty). It cuts out the soft palate tissues behind the hard palate, and many surgeons from years gone by (less so nowadays) hail this surgery as the cure for snoring.

Regardless of what UPPP does for snoring, snoring is the tip of an iceberg in most patients. Now that we measure respiration more carefully with advanced devices (pressure transducers), we rarely see cases of snoring only. Most suffer from UARS. Therefore, does UPPP cure UARS or sleep apnea? As often as not, the procedure has little to no clinically meaningful impact on the Respiratory Disturbance Index. More importantly, a bit of emerging evidence suggests that by removing the soft palate, PAP therapy becomes more difficult to attempt, because the soft palate is no longer there to guide airflow toward the back of the throat, or the back of the nasopharynx may become more constricted (stenosis). What's particularly disturbing about this surgical approach is that many surgeons still do not inform their patients of the necessity to obtain a sleep study before and after surgery to document SDB severity and changes.

When your sleep is broken, you must test your sleep objectively before and after someone conducts surgery on your body, when the alleged reason for the surgery was to fix your sleep.

Surgical Tips

Surgery has dramatic results, near-curative at times, but you want to find a surgeon affiliated with a sleep center, or who through years of experience understands the complexities of SDB and how great precision is needed to carefully tailor surgery to the individual case. Many surgical procedures are available that prove helpful, especially when performed by a physician who appreciates the goal of improving your sleep-disordered breathing but not necessarily curing it. The three most useful procedures repair a deviated septum, shrink or otherwise reduce swollen nasal turbinates, or remove tonsils and adenoids. All these procedures usually reduce the RDI or make it easier to use PAP therapy or OAT.

Surgery options should not be considered a last resort, because surgery may be a place to start for some individuals with severe or congenital malformations in their face and airway, especially among chronic mouth breathers. These sites of anatomical obstruction cause severe SDB and make OAT or PAP therapy difficult to use. So surgery on the septum, turbinates, or tonsils is worth considering. In some cases a fourth procedure, sinus surgery, may be helpful, too. But when you go down the surgical pathway, you simply want to ask your surgeon one question:

"What were the average postoperative changes in the Respiratory Disturbance Index in the last twenty-five patients for whom you have performed this surgical intervention?" And remember, RDI also includes a count of UARS events. If you want to ask one more question, you could try:

"How many of these patients, according to their sleep specialists, were able to use PAP therapy more effectively following surgery?"

Answers to these two questions will help you find the best sleep surgeon.

Other Sleep Disorders

Other sleep disorders may be a component of your overall disturbance, and no small number of patients will be afflicted with central sleep apnea problems combined with their obstructive breathing events. In addition, such things as sleepwalking or sleep-wake schedule irregularities (circadian rhythm factors) frequently affect individuals with mental health concerns and sleep problems. Occasionally, sleepiness conditions enter into the equation, such as narcolepsy or unexplained hypersomnia. Neurologic conditions including sleep-related seizures or possibly injurious sleepwalking also are not uncommon.

This book has purposely avoided discussion of other disorders, because they are best investigated, diagnosed, and treated by a sleep specialist and through regular consultation at a sleep medical center. As before, many with these types of complaints often suffer sleep breathing or sleep movement problems that underlie the other disorder. Treatment of a breathing or movement condition often improves the other disorder or fully resolves it. However, for those with narcolepsy, circadian rhythm disorders, or sleep-walking, it is essential to consult with a sleep specialist sooner rather than later.

SLEEP ON IT
Summing Up

QUESTION: How can we best sum up Sleep Dynamic Therapy?

COMMENT: SDT teaches you seven key ideas to embrace and practice:

1. Recognize that *Poor Sleep Quality* is the overriding sleep problem, affecting both mind and body in ways that damage your ability to see the impact of broken sleep on your health and life.
2. Appreciate how to observe and monitor your own sleep quality, in spite of the cognitive impairment from which you suffer, to precisely analyze your sleep problems and measure your treatment progress.
3. Understand, change, and treat mental and emotional behaviors that prevent closure at the end of the day and sound sleep at night.
4. Understand, change, and treat physical conditions that prevent closure at the end of the day and restorative sleep at night.
5. Enact and sustain all such changes by learning to:
   * *think* in radically new ways about sleep;
   * *feel* in enlightened new ways by developing emotional processing skills;
   * *image* in exciting new ways by developing imagery skills.
6. Once these key abilities take root, they will help you address any remaining mental or physical conditions that block your path to *Sound Sleep*.
7. Diligence in applying these steps is crucial in the early course of treatment; and maintenance of healthy sleep habits, behaviors, and treatments is invariably a lifelong commitment.

Seven keys that undoubtedly take considerable patience, effort, and determination to learn and to apply. If not now, when?

——— PEARL ———
Sleep Dynamic Therapy Resources

Our Web site www.sleepdynamictherapy.com is interactive and supplies educational seminars and other products and services to help problematic sleepers in their quest for *Sound Sleep*. We also have developed a VIP program for individuals who want to receive care at our sleep center in New Mexico, Maimonides Sleep Arts & Sciences, Ltd.

We have programs to teach therapists how to integrate Sleep Dynamic Therapy steps into their personal and professional efforts to improve sleep in themselves and in their patients.

Our Web site www.sleeptreatment.com is for those seeking on-site treatment at our centers in New Mexico.

Our Web site www.nightmaretreatment.com is designed for special help for chronic nightmare sufferers.

Epilogue

Words of Wisdom

The Sufis say, "He who tastes, knows."

So, too, with *Sound Sleep*. Once you taste it, you see that aggressive treatment of *Poor Sleep Quality* can solve most or all your sleep disturbances. And Sleep Dynamic Therapy has provided a step-by-step program to teach you how to obtain this remarkably enhanced form of sleep quality and all its benefits.

More than ever before, you can see the value of a lifelong commitment to your sleep health. And you can join the revolution unfolding around the world in which the power of sleep medicine is becoming crystal clear in many areas of health and in life.

Imagine these remarkable occurrences, which we already see with sleep medicine treatments that transform sleep quality:

- heart patients who live longer and with better quality of life;
- reduction in strokes and diseases previously caused by high blood pressure;
- reduction in deaths due to motor vehicle crashes;
- children whose school performance jumps a full grade level;
- children who are cured of attention deficit disorders;
- trauma survivors who sleep all night without nightmares;
- real symptom change in patients with fibromyalgia or chronic fatigue;
- sustainable improvements in mental health without drugs;
- reduction in workplace accidents;

- and, perhaps the potential for one of the greatest increases in worker productivity ever recorded in human history.

Sound Sleep delivers on these prospects, in no small part due to its impact on your energy level. Yet, in our current culture, we have forgotten the true meaning of the phrase "Sleep on it," whereas within another decade or two, scientific research will be so compelling and so conclusive that it will be obvious how much our health is being destroyed by the absence of *Sound Sleep*, and how much our health can be restored by regaining *Sound Sleep*.

Once you become one of the lucky ones who experiences *Sound Sleep*, your mind and your body confidently anticipate that your overnight experience recharges your batteries to a level that helps you tackle nearly every problem you face. Not only will you be able to recharge your energy, but also your will, and ultimately your spirit, night after night, because you can experience one of life's sacred treasures, *Sound Sleep*.

We have been blessed with a psychological and physiological system that gives us the daily break we need to cope effectively with the rigors, stresses, and challenges of life.

Sleep is this system, and it can be an every-night, all-night antidote to our daily life's trials and tribulations. Still, few in modern times seem to recognize its incredible capacity to ease some of the bitterness out of the bittersweet world in which we live.

Sleep is not a panacea; it will not cure all ailments, but it is a fundamental part of nearly every aspect of your health, and it is one of your most important and reliable sources of energy.

Sound Sleep and the *Sound Mind* that follows, though, do not necessarily provide you with perfect clarity on how to use this new fount of energy. As you change into a person with greater vigor and more vitality, you must harness this energy for the greater good of yourself and of humanity.

To do so, you must learn to use this energy wisely.

Index

NOTE: Page numbers in *italics* refer to illustrations.